PSYCHOSOCIAL ASPECTS OF CHRONIC ILLNESS AND DISABILITY AMONG AFRICAN AMERICANS

Psychosocial Aspects of Chronic Illness and Disability Among African Americans

FAYE Z. BELGRAVE

AUBURN HOUSE
Westport, Connecticut • London

Library of Congress Cataloging-in-Publication Data

Belgrave, Faye Z.
Psychosocial aspects of chronic illness and disability among African Americans / Faye Z. Belgrave.
p. cm.
Includes bibliographical references and index.
ISBN 0-86569-242-4 (alk. paper)
1. Afro-Americans—Health and hygiene—Psychological aspects. 2. Afro-Americans—Health and hygiene—Social aspects. 3. Afro-Americans—Medical care—Psychological aspects. 4. Afro-Americans—Medical care—Social aspects. 5. Health services accessibility—United States. 6. Chronic diseases—Patients—Care—United States. I. Title.
RA448.5.N4B35 1998
362.1'089'96073—dc21 98-9835

British Library Cataloguing in Publication Data is available.

Library of Congress Catalog Card Number: 98-9835
ISBN 0-86569-242-4

First published in 1998

Auburn House, 88 Post Road West, Westport, CT 06881
An imprint of Greenwood Publishing Group Inc.

Printed in the United States of America

The paper used in this book complies with the Permanent Paper Standard issued by the National Information Standards Organization (Z39.48-1984).

10 9 8 7 6 5 4 3 2 1

Contents

Illustrations

TABLES

FIGURE

Acknowledgments

Several institutions and individuals contributed to this book. Dr. Sylvia Walker, Director of the Howard University Research and Training Center on Underserved Populations provided me many opportunities to conduct research on issues related to disability among African Americans. Thank you Dr. Walker for your dedicated efforts on behalf of consumers with disabilities. Appreciation is extended to the National Institute of Mental Health and the National Institute of Disability and Rehabilitation Research for funding much of my research. Several individuals contributed to projects funded by this research. They are Drs. Sonia R. Banks, Audrey Davis, L. Lisbeth Jarama, Tirsis Quesada, Tiffany G. Townsend, Maria Cecilia Zea, and Judy Vajda. Denise Hopkins and Maribel Roldan spent countless hours conducting literature reviews and providing editing assistance. Finally, but certainly not least, gratitude is extended to the thousands of consumers with disabilities who participated in research efforts. We have learned much from you to share with others.

Introduction

Disability and chronic illness affect every citizen in the United States. The pervasive and profound consequences of disability and chronic illness affect us at the individual, family, community, and societal levels. African Americans are disproportionally affected by disability and chronic illness when compared to Whites and other ethnic minority groups. Approximately one out of every seven African Americans has an impairment that affects functioning in activities of daily living. This means in reality that almost every African American is touched by disability and chronic illness through direct experience or by the disability and chronic illness of a family member. Moreover, each of us will almost certainly have a disability or chronic illness in our lifetime if we live long enough.

The presence of disability and chronic illness impacts the quality of life for all Americans. This is especially true for African Americans. However, in spite of the significant number of African Americans who are affected by chronic illnesses and disabilities, there has been limited research and writing on the topic. The purpose of this book is to contribute to an understanding of chronic illness and disability among African Americans. This book also seeks to broaden our understanding of the ways in which mental health and functional outcomes such as employment can be improved for African Americans with chronic illnesses and disabilities.

PART I: CONTEXTUAL FRAMEWORK

The three chapters in this part provide an overview of the prevalence of disabilities and chronic illnesses and explore cultural factors that impact both antecedents and outcomes for African Americans with them.

Chapter 1: Disability and Chronic Illness Among African Americans: An Overview

The chapter begins with definitions of and distinctions between impairment, chronic illness, and disability. The status of African Americans with chronic illnesses and disabilities is presented next in this chapter. Statistical data from the National Health Interview Survey and other sources are provided to inform the reader of the extent of disability and chronic illness among African Americans (Centers for Disease Control and Prevention [CDC], 1994). These data compare the prevalence and incidence of disease, disability, and morbidity of African Americans and Whites.

This chapter also provides a snapshot of African Americans with disabilities. Data pertaining to gender, income, educational level, employment status, and other characteristics of this population are reviewed.

Chapter 2: Health, Medical, and Rehabilitation Utilization Patterns: Cultural Considerations

A primary reason for increased disability and chronic illness among African Americans is that African Americans, compared to Whites, are less likely to use medical and rehabilitation services. Information on health, medical, and rehabilitation utilization patterns is provided in this chapter. Some of the author's work on differences in rehabilitation utilization patterns of African Americans and Whites with disabilities is reviewed in this chapter. This chapter reviews the literature on factors that affect health care and rehabilitation utilization. These factors include access, attitudinal, and cultural factors. One contribution of this chapter is a discussion of why, even when medical, rehabilitation, and health services are available and accessible, they may not be used by African Americans.

The author's study on health-care adherence or compliance among African Americans with chronic illnesses is reviewed in this chapter. Her research identified several key factors related to health care compliance among African Americans with chronic illness. The final section of the chapter provides recommendations of strategies for increasing health care utilization.

Chapter 3: Cultural Influences on Disability and Outcomes

Culture impacts how one thinks about and experiences a chronic illness and disabling condition. The impact of culture on disability is discussed in chapter 3. Attitudes about persons with disabilities including self attitudes are shaped by one's culture. This chapter examines research on factors related to self attitudes and attitudes toward persons with disabilities.

One contribution of this chapter is that it provides an examination of Africentric beliefs and worldview (i.e., those beliefs, worldviews, and values that are central to persons of African descent). The application of this worldview provides the reader with a context for understanding how African Americans experience chronic illness and disability. Examples of how culture, values, and beliefs impact a variety of outcomes, including morbidity, health care utilization, mental health status, and so on are discussed in this chapter.

PART II: ADAPTIVE FUNCTIONING

The three chapters in this part focus on factors that contribute to successful outcomes among African Americans with disabilities and chronic illnesses. Each chapter considers antecedents and outcomes relevant to African Americans. Factors related to successful employment among African Americans is the subject of chapter 4. The role of social support in enhancing mental health and functional outcomes is discussed in chapter 5. Chapter 6 provides an examination of intrapersonal resources or cognitive factors that contribute to adaptive functioning. Each chapter considers the culture of African Americans in its discussion of adaptive and maladaptive functioning.

Chapter 4: Factors Contributing to Employment Success

Only 22% of working-age African Americans with disabilities are employed or seeking employment; only 16% are actually working. In this country, employment is a critical determinant of quality of life. Therefore, efforts to identify factors that contribute to successful employment are warranted. This is the aim of chapter 4. The author reviews some of the research she and colleagues have conducted on this important topic. The findings from this research identify several predictors of successful employment outcomes. Recommendations for improving employment outcomes are offered.

Chapter 5: The Role of Social Support in Adaptive Functioning

Social support has been linked to decreased morbidity, mortality, and generally enhanced mental and physical functioning. An understanding of social support for African Americans with disabilities and chronic illness is important. Chapter 5 focuses on the role of social support and how social support mediates outcomes for African Americans with disabilities.

The chapter provides an overview of the social support literature, including literature on social support among African Americans with disabilities. The author's research on social support and depression and functional outcomes among African Americans and Whites with disabilities is reviewed in this chapter.

Chapter 6: Intrapersonal Resources for Increasing Adaptive Functioning

One's cognitions (i.e., thoughts, beliefs, and ways of viewing the world) have a pervasive influence on behavior, including the experiencing of disabilities and chronic illnesses. These cognitions are conceptualized by the author as intrapersonal resources insofar as they allow us to use inner resources to help us function competently. Chapter 6 provides an examination of two intrapersonal resources as they impact functional and mental health outcomes for African Americans with chronic illnesses and disabilities. These are (a) self-efficacy and other types of psychological control and (b) coping strategies.

PART III: CULTURALLY CONGRUENT APPROACHES

This part addresses the question of what can be done to improve mental health and functional outcomes for African Americans with disabilities and chronic illnesses. Two chapters in this section are devoted to addressing this issue. One chapter focuses on how to enhance external/environmental resources (social support), and one focuses on how to enhance intrapersonal resources (i.e., self-efficacy beliefs and feelings of control).

The strategies and interventions reviewed in these chapters are based on the work of the author and her colleagues. Guidelines for implementing a social support intervention (chapter 7) and guidelines for implementing a self-efficacy intervention (chapter 8) are provided. Chapter 9 provides a conclusion to the book and discusses areas where future work is needed.

Chapter 7: Implementing a Social Support Intervention

Programs and strategies that teach individuals to identify, access, and use supportive relationships may be beneficial. Chapter 7 provides guidelines on how to design, develop, and implement a social support intervention for African Americans with chronic illnesses and disabilities. The guidelines provided in this chapter are culturally congruent and take into consideration core Africentric values. Several topics are covered in this chapter including (a) how to identify and convene group participants, (b) the role of the group leader or facilitator; and (c) the structuring of sessions. This chapter also provides an outline for a seven-session social support group intervention.

Chapter 8: Empowering African Americans Through Perceptions of Control and Self-efficacy Beliefs

Strategies for increasing self-efficacy are discussed in chapter 8. Many of these strategies were used in an intervention program that was successfully implemented by the author and colleagues. These strategies are considered empowering insofar as they can be developed from within the individual. Chapter 8 also provides a discussion of secondary control or control strategies that can be used when the individual cannot personally achieve desired outcomes. Spirituality is also discussed.

Chapter 9: Conclusions and Directions for Future Work

Chapter 9 provides a summary of major themes throughout the book and delineates areas where future programmatic and research efforts are needed.

PART I

Contextual Framework

1

Disability and Chronic Illness Among African Americans: An Overview

About 35 million Americans (about one in seven) have a disabling condition that affects functioning in activities of daily living (Institute of Medicine [IOM], 1991). About 9 million Americans are prevented from working, attending school, or maintaining a household because of a physical or mental condition. These figures reflect the certainty that disability affects every individual and family within communities, work environments, schools, and other institutions in this country. In spite of the high prevalence and incidence of disability in this country, relatively little has been written about African Americans with disabilities.

Disability and chronic illness have enormous health, social, economic, vocational, educational, and psychological consequences for everyone. This is especially true for African Americans. Often well-being and quality of life for these Americans are compromised by a disability or chronic illness. However, chronic illness and disability do not have to be associated with negative outcomes. Suggestions and recommendations for improving the well-being of African Americans with disabilities and chronic illnesses are offered throughout.

DEFINITIONS

Chronic illnesses are typically diseases that cannot be cured but can be managed by the individual. The prevalence of chronic diseases (e.g., cancer, heart disease, diabetes) is high in this country, with a substantial number of working-age persons having at least one chronic condition. About 80% of the elderly have a chronic condition (IOM, 1991). Chronic disease often increases the probability of having a disability, although disability does not necessarily occur with chronic illness. Problems associated with chronic illnesses may arise as a result of the illness itself and/or as a consequence of the treatment. Chronic illnesses are likely to affect all aspects of a person's life because of the episodic and recurring nature of symptoms. Problems are not limited to physical problems but may also occur within the vocational domain and within social and interpersonal relationships. Intrapersonal or psychological problems may also arise from the chronic illness. However, poor vocational, social, and intrapersonal outcomes are not inevitable, as many individuals are able to adapt to and cope successfully with a chronic illness. In this book, reasons for successful and not so successful coping among African Americans with chronic illnesses are explored.

A *disability* is defined primarily as a limitation in performing certain roles and tasks that society expects of an individual (IOM, 1991). Expected roles and tasks are defined by cultural norms. For example, in this country, society expects a 35-year-old male to be employed in a job outside the home. A 15-year-old male is expected to be in school. When these roles cannot be performed because of a physical or psychiatric limitation, the individual is considered disabled. Thus, the expression of a disability is socially and contextually defined. The interaction of the person's limitation within his or her social and physical environment determines whether a disability is expressed. If the environment (both physical and nonphysical) is supportive of the individual, a disability may not be experienced.

A disability may result from an impairment and/or a functional limitation. An *impairment* is an individual's loss of a mental, physiological, or biochemical function or abnormalities in these functions. Examples include having a stroke, heart attack, broken limb, or ulcers. An impairment, such as a stroke, can contribute to a functional limitation. For example, when a person has a stroke, there may be some limitation in mobility. However, impairments do not necessarily lead to functional limitations. An individual with ulcers may not be functionally limited if the condition is appropriately treated. Moreover, impairments may lead to functional limitations in some, but not all areas or domains. For example, a person who has had a stroke may be functionally limited in her ability to walk. However, this person may not be limited in other areas (e.g., communication skills).

Even when there is a functional limitation, a disability may not occur. A person who lectures for a living, for example, may not be disabled at work if she has a mobility limitation. On the other hand, an individual who is mobility impaired and employed in a job in which mobility is required would have a disability. In this context, *disability* is defined as the absence of needed environmental resources that are not available to the individual.

The extent to which an impairment such as a chronic illness becomes a functional limitation or disability depends on the facilitative and inhibitory factors within the person's environment. For example, an individual who uses a wheelchair would not necessarily be functionally impaired and/or have a disability if there was a supportive architectural environment for wheelchair users within the person's home, community, and place of employment. A person who is deaf would not necessarily be disabled if her social environment consisted of individuals who could communicate in sign language. Many of the problems faced by African Americans with disabilities are in part due to the lack of a supportive environment.

Environmental resources (both physical and nonphysical) are limited within many African American communities. This may in part be due to socioeconomic factors, including lack of employment opportunities, limited access to social services and health agencies, and the presence of environmental stressors, but the lack of physical and material resources are not the only contributing factors. Social factors and cultural beliefs also contribute to a supportive or unsupportive environment.

Intrapersonal factors also contribute to whether an impairment is expressed as a functional limitation or disability. *Intrapersonal factors* may include beliefs, thoughts, feelings, and cognitions used by individuals to organize, think about, and view themselves and the world. For example, a person with a high degree of optimism and self-efficacy is likely to seek out and engage in activities that promote lower levels of impairment and disability. This individual is likely to persevere under conditions of adversity and setbacks and seek out treatment and therapeutic regimens to improve functioning. The more optimistic and self-efficacious persons will ultimately have less disability. The worldviews and beliefs of African Americans can both facilitate and inhibit successful coping with a disability or chronic illness.

SCOPE OF THE PROBLEM

Chronic Disease Among African Americans

Statistics on the prevalence of chronic conditions among African Americans were obtained from the National Health Interview Survey. This survey included a random sample of African Americans. Data were collected from 1986–1990 (Centers for Disease Control and Prevention [CDC], 1994). The age-adjusted prevalence of the leading chronic con-

Table 1.1
Prevalence for Selected Chronic Conditions for African American and White Men and Women, 1986–1990

Conditions	Females African American %	Females White %	Males African American %	Males White %
Hypertension	19.73	10.96	13.79	10.32
Asthma	5.07	4.30	4.43	4.26
Diabetes	4.89	2.36	4.13	2.45
Chronic bronchitis	4.02	6.23	2.88	4.42
Ischemic heart disease	1.42	1.83	1.64	3.53
Stroke	1.20	0.98	1.54	1.14
Emphysema	0.17	0.58	0.93	1.21
Liver diseases	-	-	0.33	0.26

Note: From Centers for Disease Control and Prevention, *Chronic Disease in Minority Populations* (1994), National Health Interview Survey, 1986–1990. National Center for Chronic Disease Prevention and Health Promotion, U.S. Department of Health and Human Services.

ditions among African Americans and Whites are shown in Table 1.1. African Americans report the same leading chronic conditions as Whites. However, prevalence for some chronic conditions are much higher. Hypertension and diabetes are among the most common self-reported chronic conditions among African Americans, particularly among African American women. African Americans are significantly more likely than Whites to have hypertension. Hypertension is a major risk factor for many other chronic conditions, including cardiovascular disease, diabetes, and stroke. The prevalence of hypertension is almost double for African American women compared to White women and about 34% higher for African American men than White men.

African American men and women also have a significantly higher prevalence of diabetes, as shown in Table 1.1. Asthma and stroke prevalence rates are also higher for African Americans as compared to Whites. African Americans have the highest cancer incidence of any racial or ethnic group in the United States. The incidence of cancer among African American men is about 525 per 100,000 compared to White men, who have about 450 per 100,000 cases. The age-adjusted incidence rates for all cancer sites combined was 20% higher for African American men than for White men. The cancer rates among African American women and White women are about the same, 325/100,000 and 340/100,000, respectively. However, the prognosis for cancer is poorer for African Americans when compared to that of Whites. For example, the 1983–1989 five-year relative survival rate for all cancer sites combined was 39% for African Americans and 55% for Whites. The lower survival rates for African Americans are in part attributable to delay in seeking treatment and less adequate preventive care. For example, African American women, regardless of their income, are about half as likely as White women to receive mammograms (Burns, 1997).

Functional Limitations and Disability

Who are African Americans with disabilities? Of the estimated 13.4 million working-age adults with a disability, approximately 2.4 million, or 18%, are African Americans, although African Americans comprise only 12% of the population. This represents approximately 14% of African Americans in the 16–64 year age group (Asbury et al., 1991; Bowe, 1991). These figures underscore the fact that a substantial percentage of African Americans have a disability. At a practical level, this means that almost all African American families are affected by disability. Among African Americans with a disability, 54.5% are female and 45.5% are male. The higher incidence among African American women relative to men may reflect a high self-reporting of disability or the presence of additional risk factors that contribute to disability. Seventy-two percent of all African Americans with a disability have a severe disability (Walker et al., 1996). Approximately 24.4%, or 1.8 million, of the working-age population with severe disabilities are African Americans, again reflecting a substantially higher incidence among African Americans. These figures reflect the fact that African Americans who have disabilities are much more likely to be functionally disabled, that is, not able to work, attend school, take care of a household, or participate in community activities.

Data on activity limitation and disability are obtained from the National Health Interview Survey. Activity limitation denotes a restriction in the ability to perform an activity of daily living and to fulfill roles in several areas. Statistics on activity limitations for African Americans and Whites are shown in Table 1.2 (CDC, 1994). African Americans are slightly more likely to report limitations in activity than Whites (15.9% versus 15.1%). However, at the more severe level of activity limitations, African Americans report many more limitations—6.6% of African Americans and 4.3% of Whites report being unable to carry on an activity.

It is of particular interest to examine work disability prevalence, as employment is key to quality of life. Employment is associated with both tangible (housing, shelter, medical needs) and intangible (esteem, social status, success or failure) rewards in the United States. African Americans have higher rates of unemployment within the general population as well as within the population of individuals with disabilities. Individuals are classified as having a work disability if they have a health prob-

Table 1.2
Limitations of Activity Caused by Chronic Health Condition

	African Americans %	Whites %
Total with any limitation of activity	15.9	15.1
Persons limited, but not in a major activity	3.8	5.0
Persons limited in amount or kind of major activity	5.5	5.8
Persons unable to carry on an activity	6.6	4.3

Note: From L. L. Hornor, *Black Americans: A Statistical Sourcebook* (1995). Palo Alto, CA: Information Publications.

lem or disability which prevents them from working or limits the kind or amount of work they can do. Work disability prevalence is based on individuals of working age (between the ages of 16–64.)

As seen in Table 1.3, 13.8% of African Americans (or about one in seven) self-report being work disabled, compared to 8.7% of Whites. The prevalence rates of work disability are greater for African Americans than Whites at every age level. The difference is especially salient for those in the 45–54 age range, where African Americans are almost twice as likely as Whites to be work disabled. About one in five African Americans within this age range are work disabled, compared to about 11% of Whites. African Americans who are work disabled are more likely than Whites to receive food stamps and Medicaid and to reside in public and subsidized housing (see Table 1.4). These figures reflect the dependence of African Americans on governmental subsidies to meet basic survival needs.

Education, Employment, and Income Among African Americans with Disabilities

African Americans with disabilities are not likely to be employed. Only about 13% of working-age African Americans with a disability are employed, leaving the rest either unemployed or not in the labor force (i.e., not seeking work) (Bowe, 1991; Walker et al., 1996). As noted, lack of employment has enormous implications for the individual's ability to fulfill his or her roles.

African Americans with disabilities are likely to be single. Sixty-one percent of males and 71% of females are not married. About 27% of males and 43% of females have less than 12 years of formal education. Lack of education contributes to inability to obtain employment. Low levels of education and unemployment naturally exacerbate a cycle of poverty. Forty-one percent of African Americans with a disability live on or below poverty income (Walker et al., 1996). These statistics indicate

Table 1.3
Selected Characteristics of Persons with a Work Disability, 1992

Work Disabled as a Percent of the Total Population	African Americans %	Whites %
Age Groups		
Total persons	13.8	8.7
16-24 years old	5.2	3.6
25-34 years old	10.4	5.8
35-44 years old	12.6	7.7
45-54 years old	20.1	10.8
55-64 years old	34.7	20.6

Note: From L. L. Hornor, (1995). *Black Americans: A Statistical Sourcebook*. Palo Alto, CA: Information Publications.

that African Americans with disabilities are at increased risk for stressors associated with low socioeconomic status.

Mortality Among African Americans

As expected on the basis of statistics reviewed thus far, there is increased mortality for African Americans compared to Whites. Increased mortality co-occurs with the increased prevalence of chronic conditions and disability. For example, as noted previously, the five-year survival rate for cancer is much lower for African Americans than Whites.

African Americans have excess death because of seven conditions. *Excess deaths* are defined as the number of deaths among minorities that would not have occurred had mortality rates for minorities equaled that of nonminorities. These conditions are (1) heart disease and stroke; (2) homicide and accidents; (3) cancer; (4) infant mortality; (5) cirrhosis; (6) diabetes; and (7) AIDS (U.S. Department of Health and Human Services, 1986).

What is common to all of the above conditions is that they are sometimes linked to behavioral or lifestyle factors. Excess death could be reduced if behavioral changes were made. The intent in this chapter is to highlight these differences so that the discrepancies can begin to be addressed.

Why Are There Increased Morbidity, Disability, and Mortality Among African Americans?

Several factors contribute to increased morbidity, disability, and mortality among African Americans. These factors have cultural, psycholog-

Table 1.4
Work-disabled Individuals Receiving Assistance

	African Americans %	Whites %
Receiving Social Security	28.2	28.3
Receiving Food Stamps	39.1	19.1
Covered by Medicaid	47.1	25.6
Residing in Public Housing	12.1	3.2
Residing in Subsidized Housing	7.1	3.2

Note: From L. L. Hornor, (1995). *Black Americans, A Statistical Sourcebook*. Palo Alto, CA: Information Publications.

ical, environmental, and—perhaps more speculatively—physiological origin.

Role of Stress. A voluminous amount of literature provides evidence of the negative impact of stress on immune functioning and the implication of stress in many diseases of the immune system and other systems of the body, among them cardiovascular disease, cancer, and HIV progression (Anderson, Kiecolt-Glaser, & Glaser, 1994) (Maier, Watkins, & Flesher, 1994).

Stress affects the immune system through several mechanisms. One mechanism is through behavior. Under conditions of high stress, there may be reduced attention to health behaviors, such as exercise, appropriate diet, and regular preventive medical checkups. Individuals under stress may also be less likely to comply with needed medical appointments. At a cognitive level, stress causes resources normally used in activities of daily living to be diverted; individuals experiencing stress do not think about, purposefully activate, or devote their cognitive resources to health behaviors.

Physiologically, stress alters immune functioning by reducing the number of T cells, which protect the body against disease and infection. African Americans who experience high levels of stress are at elevated risk.

Many African Americans live and work under conditions of high environmental stress. High levels of unemployment and underemployment, job-related problems, financial and economic problems, and racism are sources of increased environmental stress for African Americans (Anderson, 1991). Unemployment in particular is a major stressor for African Americans. The unemployment rate for the general African American population is considerably higher than for Whites. The unemployment rate for African Americans with disabilities is high, with the vast majority not working.

Racism is also a major stressor for many African Americans, and researchers report a correlation between racism as a stressor and negative mental and physical outcomes (Landrine & Klonoff, 1995). Such stress can lead to other conditions, including drug abuse and mental illness, which exacerbate one's likelihood of being disabled and functionally impaired. Landrine and Klonoff found that increased drug use was associated with the perception of racism.

The overt racial tension and animosity between African Americans and Whites in the recent past may also be contributing to the perception of racism. This tension has been heightened by several recently publicized incidents (e.g., the O. J. Simpson trial, the Rodney King incident, among others). In addition, new governmental policies are perceived by some African Americans as oppressive (e.g., repeal of affirmative action programs, welfare reform, etc.). These perceptions of racism (whether accurate or not) create additional stress. Finally, living and working in urban environments, where there are higher levels of crime and drug activity, contribute to stress (Phillips, 1996). African Americans are more likely to live in urban than rural or suburban environments. The stressors faced by African Americans without disabilities are magnified for African Americans with disabilities. These Americans are more likely to face stress due to economic hardship, living and working in an architecturally unsupportive environment, and stigmatization based on race as well as disability. Lack of access to medical and rehabilitation services is another major contributor to increased morbidity among African Americans.

Access Factors. Access to preventive services (e.g., regular mammograms) and treatment is hindered by poor economic conditions. Lower rates of employment and underemployment for African Americans result in less medical coverage because health insurance is not available. Even if available, health insurance subsidies may be inadequate. African Americans may be less likely to go for routine and preventive treatment because of several other access factors. These may include limited transportation, lack of money to pay for medication or therapeutic treatment, and inconvenient location of clinics/facilities. Concurrently, even when medical care and treatment are accessible for African Americans, less attention may be devoted to preventive care against the backdrop of the many other problems and concerns faced by African Americans.

Statistics show that African Americans are less likely than Whites to visit physicians and engage in routine medical care. As seen in Table 1.5, African Americans on average have 5.2 physician visits a year, compared to 5.8 for Whites. However, when hospitalized, African Americans are more likely to have a longer length of stay than Whites (see Table 1.6). This suggests that African Americans may be sicker and have more se-

Table 1.5
Characteristics of Physician Visits, 1991

Physician visit by site of visit	African Americans %	Whites %
All physicians visits (per person)	5.2	5.8
At doctor's offices	52.0	60.1
At hospital outpatient department	21.2	13.0
By telephone	7.3	12.8
Home	3.6	2.6
Other	15.8	11.5

Note: From L. L. Hornor, (1995). *Black Americans: A Statistical Sourcebook*. Palo Alto, CA: Information Publications.

vere health conditions when they go to the hospital. The role of access factors will be discussed in greater detail in chapter 2.

Cultural beliefs and worldviews also play a role in morbidity and disability impairment. Beliefs about the etiology of a particular condition may impact whether treatment is sought. For example, belief that one's well-being is determined by fate may affect the decision not to seek treatment and/or rehabilitation because of the acceptance of what is meant to be. The emphasis on communal relationships and interdependence may also prevent people from taking the time to engage in preventive health care and treatment if others are negatively affected by these actions. The facilitative and inhibitory roles of cultural factors on disability and illness will be discussed in greater detail in chapter 3.

Another reason for the increased morbidity of African Americans is that they are more likely to work under conditions in which they are at increased risk for injury and/or environmental health hazards. African Americans, compared to Whites, are more likely to be employed at low-skilled jobs where there is increased potential for accidents and injury.

An additional contributor to morbidity is residence in high-crime areas. Many African Americans live in inner-city neighborhoods besieged by crime and drugs. The violence associated with the drug trade in many of our inner-city neighborhoods leads to increased levels of trauma, including brain injuries and spinal cord injuries, especially among young African American males.

SUMMARY

In overview, African Americans are at increased risk for chronic illnesses and disability because of several factors. The prevalence of disability is quite high within the African American community, and the outcomes for African Americans with disabilities are fairly poor. About one out of seven working-age African Americans has a disabling con-

Table 1.6
Hospital Short Stays: Discharges, Days of Care, and Average Length of Stay for African Americans and Whites, 1992

	African Americans	Whites
Discharges	106.6	87.8
Days of care	736.0	547.2
Average length of stay	6.9	6.2

Note: From L. L. Hornor, (1995). *Black Americans: A Statistical Sourcebook.* Palo Alto, CA: Information Publications.

dition that limits functioning in activities of daily living. The vast majority of African Americans with disabilities are not employed, many are poor, and many live in environments in which there is little support. Yet the outcomes of African Americans with disabilities are not invariably negative. A supportive environment and intrapersonal resources make it possible for African Americans with chronic illnesses and disabilities to lead successful, productive lives.

2

Health, Medical, and Rehabilitation Utilization Patterns: Cultural Considerations

Disparities in morbidity, mortality, and disability among African Americans and other ethnic groups were discussed in chapter 1. As noted there, a substantial percentage of African Americans are disabled and have functional impairments that impact their ability to function at home, at work, and within the community. Health, medical, and utilization patterns of African Americans account in part for these disparities. The differing utilization patterns are influenced by economical, psychological, social, and cultural factors. The contributions of utilization patterns to disability and functioning among African Americans are discussed in this chapter. This chapter is divided into four sections. In the first section, statistics on utilization of health, medical, and rehabilitation services and programs among African Americans are reviewed. The second section of this chapter focuses on factors that affect health, medical, and rehabilitation utilization. Health care adherence, the degree to which health or medical recommendations are followed, is closely related to utilization and will be discussed in the third section. The author's research on compliance among African Americans with chronic illnesses will be discussed in this section. The fourth section provides strategies for increasing health, medical, and rehabilitation utilization.

HEALTH AND MEDICAL UTILIZATION PATTERNS

Utilization of health and medical services is lower for African Americans than Whites across several domains. As noted in the previous chapter, African Americans have fewer physician contacts per year than White Americans. However, when African Americans do get sick, they tend to become sicker than Whites. This is reflected in the fact that hospital outpatient visits (usually visits to the emergency room) by African Americans exceed those of White Americans. The length of stay per hospital visit is also greater for African Americans than White Americans (see Tables 1.4 and 1.5 in chapter 1). These disparities can, in part, be accounted for by the lack of routine and preventive health care for African Americans. These statistics suggest that many African Americans are not obtaining routine and preventive care and that hospital emergency rooms are being used to replace routine physician contact.

Rehabilitation Service Utilization

The underutilization of services is also seen in the rehabilitation arenas. Ethnic minorities are less likely to participate in state vocational rehabilitation programs and to be successfully rehabilitated (Walker, Asbury, Rodriguez, & Saravonabhauer, 1996). This is a disturbing trend, given that disability is more pronounced among African Americans, and functional outcomes are less favorable. Rehabilitation, to date, remains the most viable mechanism by which optimal functioning can be restored or facilitated. Yet African Americans do not benefit from rehabilitation to the extent that they could or should.

Study on Rehabilitative Service Utilization Patterns. In this study, Belgrave and Walker (1991a) examined differences between African Americans and White Americans regarding utilization of rehabilitation services. A nonrandom sample of 170 African Americans and 45 White Americans was selected from the client rosters at rehabilitation agencies that participated in the study. These public and private rehabilitation agencies were in the eastern, western, and midwestern regions of the United States and selected because they were in cities that had a sizable ethnic minority population.

An overview of the demographic characteristics of African American and White American participants is shown in Table 2.1. As seen in the table, the two ethnic groups were quite similar on most demographic characteristics. The majority of participants in both groups were unemployed, single, and had income derived from employment of less than $5,000. Regarding coverage for health and medical services, the majority

Table 2.1
Characteristics of Participants in Rehabilitation Service Utilization Study

	African Americans	Whites
Age		
Mean	44.5	43.2
Range	21-82	21-83
	%	%
Gender		
Female	47.3	57.8
Male	52.7	42.2
Marital status		
Married	24.4	22.2
Single	64.9	75.6
Widowed	10.7	2.2
Educational level		
< H.S	44.8	34.1
≥ H.S.	55.2	65.9
Employment		
Employed	20.2	22.2
Not employed	78.8	77.8
Income		
< $5,000	55.0	50.0
$5,000 - 10,000	7.0	10.0
$10,000 - 20,000	20.0	13.3
> $20,000	8.0	26.7

of participants from both groups had Medicaid, 52.3% and 57.5% for African Americans and Whites, respectively.

Participation in rehabilitation programs was assessed via a self-report questionnaire. Participants were asked to indicate if they were currently receiving rehabilitation services in the areas of (a) physical therapy, (b) occupational therapy, (c) vocational rehabilitation, and (d) counseling.

Table 2.2 shows the percentage of African Americans and White Americans receiving services in each of the rehabilitation service categories. Chi-square analyses were performed to determine whether the reported differences were statistically significant.

The chi-square revealed large and significant differences between African Americans and White Americans across several rehabilitation services. African Americans were less likely than Whites to report receiving physical therapy ($p < .001$). Twice as many Whites as African Americans

Table 2.2
African Americans and Whites with Disabilities Who Participate in Rehabilitation Services

	African Americans	Whites
Physical therapy	20.0	40.9
Occupational therapy	2.9	34.1
Counseling	20.0	45.5
Vocational rehabilitation	31.2	29.5

reported they were currently in physical therapy (41% versus 20%). Ten times more Whites than African Americans reported being in an occupational therapy program (34% versus 3%). This difference was significant ($p < .001$). Finally, more than twice as many Whites as African Americans reported receiving counseling services ($p < .001$) (46% versus 20%). There were no significant differences in the percentages of African Americans and Whites who were receiving vocational rehabilitation. This may be related to the fact that our sample was recruited primarily from agencies that provided vocational rehabilitation services.

Because the sample in this study was not a national probability sample, the generality of the findings should be interpreted with some caution. Nonetheless, the figures in Table 2.2 reveal some striking differences between the two groups. Across three of the four categories, the disparities were very large regarding rehabilitation participation of African Americans and White Americans.

While the data from the Belgrave and Walker (1991a) study are now somewhat outdated, Walker et al. (1996) confirmed this finding in a later study that also pointed to differences in rehabilitation utilization across ethnic groups. Findings from this study revealed that Whites and Asians have more money spent on them for rehabilitation services than African Americans and Latinos.

One plausible reason that differences might exist between African Americans and Whites in the study conducted by Belgrave and Walker is that there were socioeconomic differences between the two groups. That is, Whites were perhaps in a better position than African Americans to afford rehabilitation services. However, in looking at the demographic characteristics of the two groups shown in Table 2.1, the two groups were fairly similar—on a whole, both groups were of low socioeconomic status.

Another plausible explanation might be that there were differences between the two groups regarding health or medical coverage. That is, Whites may have had better insurance to pay for rehabilitation services than African Americans. However, this interpretation is also not plausible. The majority of participants in both ethnic groups had Medicaid (53% for African Americans and 58% for whites). While a larger percentage of Whites than African Americans reported having private insurance, 35% versus 26%, this difference is not very large. Thus the socioeconomic factors and health and medical insurance do not seem to account for the differences in rehabilitation utilization patterns. Clearly there are other factors that must account for these differences.

FACTORS RELATED TO UTILIZATION PATTERNS

Economic factors do not seem to account singularly for disparities between African Americans and Whites in medical and rehabilitation utilization patterns. In this section several factors related to health, medical, and rehabilitation utilization among African Americans are discussed. These factors help to account for the differentials in health care just discussed.

Access Factors

Access factors are concerned with whether medical care and rehabilitation services are affordable and available when needed. Additional access factors center around whether the facilities are convenient to the consumer, whether the operating hours are convenient, and whether there is accessible transportation to the facility.

Affordability can facilitate or impede access. About 30% of African Americans have incomes below the poverty level, and African Americans are twice as likely as their White counterparts to be below poverty level (U.S. Department of Health and Human Services, 1990). African Americans with disabilities are even more likely to live in poverty. A large majority do not have health coverage for acute medical needs, much less for rehabilitation services. As noted, lack of health coverage and access to a primary physician contribute to overutilization of emergency room services in the absence of routine and preventive health care.

The lack of adequate health insurance is directly related to fewer employment opportunities for African Americans generally and African Americans with disabilities specifically. African Americans with disabilities have the least favorable employment record of any ethnic group. Only a small percentage of African Americans with disabilities (16%) are employed. When employed, they are more likely to work in semiskilled and unskilled jobs that may not provide health insurance.

Thus there is a cyclical relationship between health insurance and employment. Inadequate access to rehabilitation services restricts the consumer's ability to receive services to restore maximal functioning, and this in turn limits employment opportunities. Being unemployed with no or restricted health insurance restricts participation in a health care system which could restore one to maximal functioning.

Another access barrier is lack of transportation to medical or rehabilitation facilities. In the study discussed earlier on rehabilitation service utilization patterns among African Americans and Whites, significantly more Whites than African Americans reported owning or having access to a private car or vehicle to transport them to rehabilitation appointments. African Americans were more likely to report that they used public transportation to attend medical and rehabilitation appointments. Lack of transportation can be a major access barrier for persons with disabilities.

Buses and trains are often not accessible for persons in wheelchairs and others who may need special equipment. Access to public transportation is often limited in inner cities, where many African Americans reside. Within those communities, the strong political and economic power from citizens to demand accessible and reliable public transportation services is often lacking.

Thus it is often easier for the consumer simply not to go to medical and rehabilitation appointments rather than to hassle with transportation barriers. This short-term decision has negative long-term effects; the relationship between rehabilitation participation and lack of transportation is circular. Lack of transportation prevents the individual from receiving appropriate medical and rehabilitation services. The absences of these services, in turn, contribute to the individual's inability to maximize functioning—improved functional outcomes may contribute to better transportation access.

The importance of transportation was supported in the findings of a study by Belgrave and Walker (1991b). In this study, transportation source was the strongest contributor of employment status for African Americans with disabilities. Those individuals with access to private transportation such as cars were more likely to be employed than those without.

The salience of transportation was illustrated by an incident involving the author and an African American rehabilitation consumer. The consumer was invited to participate in a program designed to improve employment potential. The program was implemented at a facility within the community. In spite of this, one person called to report that she was unable to attend the first session because she did not have money to catch a bus, and she was unable to walk the mile or so because of her disability. When told that bus tokens for transportation would be provided if she could get to the facility, she replied that she did not even have the limited few dollars needed to pay the one-way fare. This incident demonstrates that even when rehabilitation services are available and desired, there may be simple but powerful inhibitory factors.

Location of Facility. A related access problem is location of the treatment facility. Clinics, hospitals, social service agencies, rehabilitation agencies, and other facilities are often not located within communities or in close proximity to where African Americans live. Thus, travel to and from facilities may take much effort, even when private and public transportation are available.

The importance of placing programs in the community where consumers reside was illustrated in a rehabilitation program implemented by the author and colleagues. Consumers were invited to participate in a program designed to improve employment outcomes. Sessions were held in a downtown location that staff thought was accessible by public transportation. In spite of this, consumer attendance was sporadic. In discussing the low attendance problem with consumers, it became apparent that the location of the program was an inhibiting factor to participation. Sessions started early in the morning, and most of the participants had to travel for about two hours and change two buses to get to the sessions on time. This meant that they had to leave their homes as early as 7:00 A.M. to arrive at a 9:00 A.M. session. When the sessions were located within the community, (and traveling time was decreased to under 30 minutes), participation increased dramatically.

The above anecdotes illustrate the importance of being familiar with the socioenvironmental context of consumers. These anecdotes highlight the importance of ongoing communication with consumers in order to understand their needs and how these needs interact with their utilization of rehabilitation services.

Moreover, there are symbolic, as well as practical, considerations for locating services within the community where people reside. Consumers may rightly question why they have to leave their communities in order to receive adequate health and rehabilitation services. Locating programs and services within the community conveys sensitivity to and collaboration with the consumer. In the above situation, the burden was placed on program staff, not the consumer, to travel to program sites. An alternative approach is to hire persons from the community to provide health and rehabilitation services whenever possible.

Staffing and Operation of Facility. Another consideration is the accessibility of medical and rehabilitation personnel once the consumer arrives at the facility. When consumers arrive at a facility and are subject to long waiting periods and a waiting area that is crowded and unattractive, frustration results. Add to this impatience from staff overburdened with large caseloads, and negative feelings and perceptions from both health care provider and consumer will slow and disrupt the treatment experience. Unfortunately, incidents of disrespectful treatment by medical and rehabilitation personnel are all too frequent. The lack of respect is often exaggerated when the individual has no private medical coverage and the person is made to feel that he/she has no right to treatment and services. One suggestion is that consumers be trained in what to expect from health care and rehabilitation providers. Consumers need to know how to request professional and courteous services and what to do if these services are not forthcoming.

Another access factor is operating hours. Most facilities close at 5:00 or 6:00 P.M., and it may be difficult for individuals who work, do child care, or have primary responsibility for young children to attend the facility before it closes. Some evening and weekend hours are needed.

Competition of Other Needs

Several other issues might compete in African Americans' decisions to participate or not participate in rehabilitation services. As noted in chapter 1, African Americans experience increased stress as a result of several internal and external factors (Anderson, 1991; Myers, 1983). Unemployment is high within the African American community, especially in inner cities. Many of us live in communities where there are drugs and violence. Low-income housing is often unavailable and when available, inadequate. African Americans live and function within extended families whose concerns are owned and shared by all—creating additional support, but also additional stress. When one member of the family is stressed, all members of the family become so.

Within this socioenvironmental context, more immediate concerns may take priority over long-term planning for rehabilitation and other treatment needs. Rehabilitation by its very nature involves long-term systematic planning and ongoing participation. The positive rewards from participating in a rehabilitation program do not occur overnight but may take months or even years. Yet basic survival needs—food, shelter, and safety—must be dealt with daily. Within this context, even when services are accessible, there may not be active and continual participation from African American consumers.

Racism and Attitudes of Health Care and Rehabilitation Professionals

People who work in institutions and settings that serve persons with disabilities reflect the attitudes of society. Negative attitudes and discriminatory actions toward African Americans may be at the individual, cultural, or institutional level (Jones, 1997). Subtle and institutional forms of racism contribute to lower participation in rehabilitation services among African Americans. The unavailability of treatment facilities within African American communities is an example of institutional racism that negatively affects rehabilitation utilization for African Americans.

Attitudes of the rehabilitation professionals toward African Americans may also limit rehabilitation participation by African Americans. Here, individual racism may be operative in more subtle ways through acts of differential treatment to African Americans and Whites. One of the consequences of both individual and institutional racism is that African Americans may not be appropriately referred and when referred, not encouraged to remain in treatment.

A study by Walker, Belgrave, Roberts, and Palmer (1986) sheds some light on referral and rehabilitation service patterns for African Americans and other ethnic groups referred to state and private vocational rehabilitation programs. The findings of the study by Walker et al. suggest that the attitudes rehabilitation professionals hold may contribute to disparities in rehabilitation utilization patterns. In this study, data were obtained from 27 state and private rehabilitation agencies across 8 states representing the four geographic regions of the country. Data pertaining to referral source and rehabilitation status were available on 64,076 African Americans, 12,993 whites, and 1,122 Hispanics; 29,905 individuals were in other categories. These data were based on 1983 statistics obtained from state rehabilitation agencies.

One question the authors were interested in was whether the source of referrals for rehabilitation services was different for African Americans than for Whites. The investigators found several differences for the two groups. When looking at the welfare agency as a source of referral, of those referrals made, 66% were for Whites and 24% were for African Americans. In looking at the physician as a source of referrals, of those referrals made by physicians, 71% were for Whites and 23% were for African Americans. One would expect physicians to be good sources of referrals for both groups—yet discrepancies between the two ethnic groups were seen.

Data from this same study also revealed disparities regarding how consumers progress through the rehabilitation system. Of interest was what status the person was in when his or her file was closed or when the client exited the program. The investigators found that more African Americans were in an extended evaluation phase than Whites, 30% compared to 19%. Being in an extended evaluation status means essentially that these consumers had not received any rehabilitation services at the time they exited the system; that is, they were still at the evaluation stage. In this same study, 43% of Whites were in training at the time they exited the program; by contrast, only 36% of African Americans were in a training category. Obviously it is more desirable to be in training than extended evaluation status at exit from rehabilitation. Walker et al. (1986)

suggest that there may be some attitudinal barriers that impact referral for rehabilitation services and subsequent participation in rehabilitation programs.

The findings from this study reveal clear and startling differences in African Americans' and Whites' experience regarding rehabilitation services.

Divergent Values and Communication

Some cultural values, attitudes, and communication patterns differ for African Americans and Whites. When these differences exist, the exchange between the rehabilitation professional and the consumer may not be meaningful and productive. The African American consumer may not return for needed rehabilitation services following initial communication in which divergent cultural values lead to communication problems.

To illustrate a cultural difference between African Americans and Whites, a colleague recounts the frequent communication exchange between African American consumers and rehabilitation specialists (e.g., physical therapists, occupational therapists, speech therapists). These specialists may talk to African American consumers using a very familiar manner, that is, referring to them as John, Jim, and so on, instead of more formally as Mr. Smith, Mr. Jones, and so forth. This may be a natural way of communicating for the rehabilitation specialist, who may in fact communicate in this same manner with White consumers and may use this informality to promote (in her view) an interpersonal relationship. In fact, the African American consumer may view this lack of formality as being talked down to and find such language offensive. Being referred to by one's first name may seem disrespectful to African Americans, especially older men who were historically addressed by their first names by White persons who called them by their first name as a putdown and a way to keep them in their place.

Another turn-off is rehabilitation professionals who speak in professional or technical jargon, minimizing the consumer's ability to understand the message. Unanswered questions may remain unanswered, and the opportunity to inform and educate is lost. Similarly medical or rehabilitation professionals may talk in a manner that is condescending and patronizing. When this happens, the consumer is not viewed as an intelligent person capable of communicating his/her needs and desires.

Values and Beliefs of African Americans. African Americans also have values and beliefs that may impact rehabilitation service utilization patterns. These cultural beliefs for African Americans are rooted in West African beliefs and will be discussed in greater detail in chapter 3. For now, an illustration of how a communal and interpersonal orientation may facilitate or impede health and rehabilitation utilization may be helpful.

One Africentric dimension among African Americans is communal and relationship-orientations, in contrast to individualistic and materialistical orientations. This orientation stresses and places a positive value on the person's ability to connect with and to establish a harmonious interpersonal relationship with others. From this perspective, the ability of the provider to establish an interpersonal relationship with the consumer should facilitate the rehabilitation progress. In other words, if the person "likes" or "connects" with the consumer, rehabilitation utilization patterns should be facilitated. In this context, sincerity and genuineness are important for the provider to convey to the consumer. This orientation may be contrasted with a more Eurocentric orientation whereby perceived expertise and competency rather than interpersonal relationship may be valued. For African American consumers, having expertise and skill may not be enough and compliance to recommendations is likely to be influenced by how well the consumer likes, trusts, and respects the professional. The ways in which Africentric values and beliefs impact participation in the rehabilitation process will be discussed in greater detail in the next chapter.

A final consideration is that many African Americans simply do not trust that Whites will do what is in their best interest. This guarded suspicion is justifiable among African Americans, who have lived for hundreds of years under oppressive conditions. Therefore, no matter how well intended, the rehabilitation specialist who is White may be looked upon with some guarded suspicion.

FACTORS RELATED TO HEALTH CARE ADHERENCE AMONG AFRICAN AMERICANS WITH DISABILITIES

One aspect of health utilization is health care adherence or compliance. Health care adherence is the extent to which an individual follows medical or health recommendations in three areas: 1) keeping appointments; 2) taking medication; and 3) adhering to healthy behaviors (i.e., eating nutritiously, exercising, controlling stress, having regular blood pressure checkups, etc.). Health care adherence is an important aspect of medical and rehabilitation utilization. In fact, patterns of health care adherence may parallel those of medical and rehabilitation utilization for African Americans.

For persons with disabilities and chronic illnesses, adherence to prescribed health recommendations may not only impact the quality of their lives, but whether they live or die. For example, for some persons with diabetes, taking insulin prevents coma. For an individual who is living with AIDS, learning how to deal with stressors that can negatively impact the immune system is critical. For persons with any chronic illness or debilitating condition, regular medical appointments to follow the progression of the disease may be necessary and circumvent potential problems. For an obese person, eating the wrong foods and failure to exercise increase the risk of several diseases, including cardiovascular disease, diabetes, and cancer. As noted in chapter 1, African Americans are at increased risk for several of these diseases. Lack of adherence may be a larger concern when the individual has a chronic illness or a disability and recommendations aimed at decreasing the deleterious effects of the chronic illness and disability are not followed.

Patterns of utilization of medical and rehabilitative services among African Americans are related to health care adherence. The literature suggests there is a great deal of variability in adherence patterns and that overall adherence rates are troublesome in most populations, including African Americans. Estimates of failure to adhere to medical treatment are high (DiMatteo & DiNicola, 1982; Sackett & Snow, 1979). Between 30% and 60% of all consumers fail to take medication as prescribed. Long-term treatment for chronic illness is particularly troublesome—up to 80% of all patients fail to carry out correctly at least one component of the therapeutic regimen. In general, failure to adhere to treatment is a far greater problem than health professionals estimate (DiMatteo & DiNicola, 1982). The author has conducted research with African Americans with particular chronic illnesses, sickle cell disease and diabetes, to examine factors that contribute to adherence. About 50% of these individuals do not adhere to scheduled medical appointments. In a study by Lewis, Belgrave, and Scott (1990), several factors related to compliance among African Americans with sickle cell disease were examined. These factors were grouped into four categories as follows: (a) psychological factors, (b) family factors, (c) community factors, and (d) institutional factors.

Psychological Factors

Psychological factors such as coping ability affect health care adherence. Limited resources and a history of oppression may contribute to feelings of powerlessness and interfere with the individual's ability to cope with stress in a competent way. Given such background, some African Americans may feel powerless and hopeless regarding health and related outcomes. Consequently, individuals may not know how to optimally access and derive benefits from the health care system.

On the other hand, self-efficacious beliefs that one can overcome adversity and be restored to optimal functioning should facilitate adherence to appropriate treatment regimens. Self-efficacious beliefs also contribute to the individual's ability to identify resources that may be useful for improving adherence and rehabilitation utilization. Strategies for increasing adaptive coping and self-efficacy are discussed in Part III of this book.

Family Factors

The family may be a facilitative or inhibitory factor in health care adherence. The extended Black family is composed of multiple generations of kin and non-kin who share and support one another. Historically, the African American family has been central to African and African American life (Martin & Martin, 1978; McAdoo, 1982, 1993). Thus, the problems of one member of the family are shared by all members. When there are decisions to be made about health care utilization patterns, family members may consult each other, and the resources of the family may be shared for the good of the individual. Thus a family member is likely to baby-sit for the mother who has to attend an appointment, or a ride to an appointment may be provided.

Overreliance on the family at the expense of other systems can also have negative results. It may be important for the consumer to learn to identify resources outside the family that can be used to help one achieve desired goals. It is not likely that the family will have all necessary resources for assisting all family members in medical and rehabilitation treatment (e.g., the family may not be the best source of information about the most appropriate treatment regimen).

Community Factors

A third set of variables that impact adherence within the African American community is community variables. The community can contribute positively or negatively to health care adherence. Several support systems in the African American community may facilitate involvement in the health care systems. These support systems include neighbors, local merchants, the church, and ministers. These support systems may complement more formal social services and health care systems. For example, the Black church is a focal point in many African American communities—within the church, health, education, economic, and health agendas are discussed and promoted. It is not uncommon for African American churches to host job fairs, health fairs, and educational forums. The minister and deacons of the church frequently are leaders in the community.

In an attempt to delineate how psychological, family, community, and institutional factors impact health care adherence of African Americans with sickle cell disease, research was conducted by the author and colleagues (Belgrave & Lewis, 1994). In this study, data pertaining to appointment-keeping patterns were obtained from 70 persons attending a center for sickle cell disease. Appointment-keeping patterns were considered an important measure of adherence for persons with sickle cell disease, who may need regular follow-up appointments to monitor symptoms and overall medical and physiological indicators. Appointment-keeping behavior was assessed by asking consumers about their appointment-keeping behaviors and by reviewing medical records. An index of appointment-keeping behavior (from high to low) was derived for each person.

Measures of psychological variables (i.e., self-esteem, perceived control), community and family variables (i.e., perceived social support), and institutional variables (i.e., treatment environment) were obtained. Additionally, measures of perceived disease severity (symptom checklist, perception of disease severity) were obtained from participants along with demographic information.

A multivariate analysis (regression) was computed, with the described variables entered as explanatory (predictor) variables and appointment-keeping behavior as the outcome (dependent) variable. The results were significant and revealed that about one-fifth of the variance in appointment-keeping behavior could be explained by the factors examined in this study. Having good support from the family and the community, feeling in control of one's health, and having a treatment facility that is positively viewed were the most significant factors in appointment-keeping behavior.

The findings of the study on compliance among African Americans with sickle cell disease also illustrate the importance of utilizing a comprehensive approach for understanding and promoting health care adherence and utilization among African Americans. In this study, no factor singularly explained adherence, but several factors jointly and interactively influenced adherence for this group of African Americans.

STRATEGIES FOR INCREASING HEALTH CARE AND REHABILITATION UTILIZATION

Several strategies for increasing health and rehabilitation utilization patterns are described below. These strategies, can be implemented at the individual, family, community, and institutional level, and should also be useful for improving health care adherence.

Individual Level Strategies

Efforts to increase consumer responsibility for health and rehabilitation utilization must be directed at the individual consumer. Increasing one's beliefs that one can successfully access and participate in appropriate health and rehabilitative services should be a desired individual goal. These beliefs may be more difficult to promote among those African Americans who have not had extensive experience with taking control. However, these beliefs can be learned. (Strategies for increasing self-efficacy beliefs and the perception of control are discussed in chapter 8.)

The encouragement of appropriate beliefs and skills can be facilitated by other consumers. While rehabilitation and health professionals can facilitate this process, in order for true internalization of appropriate behaviors to occur, consumers must see (and subsequently model) the actions of similar others.

One helpful strategy is the creation of self-help consumer groups. Professionals can be helpful in this process by proving administrative support such as a place to meet and other necessary resources (i.e., transportation assistance if needed, child care, etc.), but the group should be consumer directed.

Self-help consumer groups could host sessions in which persons teach and train each other to access health care systems by sharing experiences and resources. Here, consumers could share their own experiences regarding what works and what doesn't. Sessions on how to be assertive and stand up for one's rights should be helpful. Having access to information on consumer legal rights could be shared within the context of these groups. (A more detailed discussion of how to implement a support group is provided in chapter 7.)

Health and rehabilitation professionals can be helpful in this process by communicating to consumers that they are ultimately responsible both for their health and related outcomes and for whether they receive appropriate treatment. Consumers should be encouraged to ask questions and to challenge the prescribed recommendation when they have doubts.

Family and Community-level Strategies

Health and rehabilitation professionals must recognize that the African American family, including the extended family, is an integral link to the consumer's access to rehabilitation and health systems. For example, a prescribed low fat/low salt diet may be circumvented if the household cook only prepares meals that are full of fat and salt. On the other hand, a consumer may rely upon a family member for transportation to a facility and may only be able to attend appointments when this family member is available.

Family members encourage appropriate utilization patterns when they serve as role models. African American family members serve as emotional as well as material sources of support when they lend money for a cab, take care of the children, and in general offer support. Supportive acts by the family contribute to the consumers' well-being in other ways by reassuring the individual that he or she is cared for and loved and that his or her well-being is of priority. Concrete tangible services such as a home-cooked meal, baby-sitting, and the loan of a car are especially welcomed by individuals with limited financial resources. (A more in-depth discussion of the family as a source of support among African Americans is provided in chapter 5.)

The church and friends from the church also play a facilitating role in utilization of health care services. Free health care screenings are often organized by churches with encouragement from ministers for the congregation to participate. Members of the church family may be supportive and encourage the person to take care of him/her self. When church members are sick, their names are put on a list of people who need prayers and members of the church family are asked to pray for, send cards to, and visit these individuals. Churches may also provide some financial and tangible support when needed.

In brief, the family and the community can provide important support. One way to increase utilization patterns is by encouraging and teaching the consumer to access support from the family and the community. (Strategies for accessing family and community support are discussed in chapter 7.)

Institutional Level Strategies

There are several institutional strategies that can be used to increase health care and rehabilitation utilization among African Americans. Rehabilitation and medical professionals should be sensitized to cultural issues that impact African Americans' utilization of health and rehabilitation services. For example, as noted earlier, among African Americans, it is important to establish a sincere relationship and to be able to connect to the consumer at an interpersonal level. Accordingly, programs need to be developed to train individuals in these areas.

Another way to increase beliefs about one's ability to access and receive appropriate services is by having appropriate role models at the facility. Making sure that the staff is ethnically and culturally diverse is another way to show sensitivity to culturally diverse consumers. Programs aimed at training and recruiting African Americans in health, medical, and rehabilitation careers should be implemented at the high school and college levels.

A consumer advocate (an African American with a disability) would be a good staff member to have at a treatment facility. This individual could bridge the gap between the consumer and the institutional staff. The consumer advocate could inform the consumer of how to negotiate to get the services they need. This consumer advocate could also help the treatment staff become more sensitive to the needs of consumers.

Finally the facility must be accessible. Hours of operation should be flexible. Perhaps the facility could stay open late one evening a week. Child care may be necessary for parents who have to bring their children with them to appointments. Transportation needs should be considered a necessary aspect of medical services. When possible, services should be located within the community in which consumers reside. Friendly reminders of appointments may also be helpful and convey to the consumer that his or her attendance is important.

Rehabilitation professionals also need to be aware of and ready to address core problems that impact the consumer, such as lack of adequate housing, employment, and food. It is unlikely that one institution or agency could take care of all of these problems, so services must be coordinated to avoid duplication.

SUMMARY

There are disparities between African Americans and Whites in health, medical, and rehabilitation utilization patterns. Several factors contribute to these disparities, including access factors, attitudinal barriers, and cultural differences. Strategies for improving utilization patterns and adherence can be implemented at the individual, family, community, and institutional level. Increased empowerment of African Americans for assuming responsibilities for health and related outcomes is an important first step. Additionally, use of family and community resources, including the church, should prove useful. Training of more African American consumers with disabilities and training in the area of cultural diversity should be helpful to professionals who are not African American.

3

Cultural Influences on Disability and Outcomes

The influence of culture on disability is pervasive. Culture impacts disability prevalence, how one thinks about and experiences a disabling condition, and how one functions as a result of a disabling condition. Culture may be considered the sum total of a society's customs, habits, beliefs, and values (Kroeber & Cluckholm, 1963). Beals (1967) defined culture as ideas, feelings, and practices that individuals adopt as members of a system. This system may include people, material objects, and customs. Leininger (1978) defined culture as a way of life that directs the actions and thoughts of a group of people. These thoughts and actions are pervasive and impact all aspects of life, including one's morbidity, mortality, and functioning. The assumption made in this chapter and throughout the book is that culture impacts how people react to and cope with chronic illness and disability. For African Americans, African, along with American, culture shape core values, beliefs, and behaviors.

The first section of this chapter provides an overview of the ways in which culture shapes one's beliefs and behaviors regarding health, illness, and disability. Attitudes about persons with disabilities including self attitudes is an important contributor to coping and adjustment. Attitudes and beliefs about disability as a function of culture and ethnicity are discussed in the next section. Also included in this section is a discussion of factors that influence positive attitudes toward disability and acceptance of disability among African Americans. For African Americans, Africentric beliefs provide the cultural context in which to understand the culture and behavior of African Americans. Africentric values and worldview are discussed in the third part of the chapter. The final section of the chapter is a discussion of how Africentric beliefs impact outcomes and functioning among African Americans with disabilities and chronic illnesses.

THE INFLUENCE OF CULTURE ON BELIEFS ABOUT HEALTH, ILLNESS, AND DISABILITY

In a discussion of culture and health schemas, Landrine and Klonoff (1992) provide a review of how culture influences health-related schemas. While much of Landrine and Klonoff's review is centered around the influence of culture on health, illness, and disease, the literature can be extended to disability and chronic illness.

In this review, Landrine and Klonoff analyze how culture influences health and illness schemas of ethnic and cultural groups in the United States and other countries and how the schemas of non-Whites differ from those of White Americans. A schema is an organized collection of beliefs or information about someone or something (Fisk & Taylor, 1991). An illness schema is an organized collection of beliefs about illness, whereas a disability schema would include organized beliefs and ways of thinking about disability or a particular type of disability. Schemas develop within and are a product of one's culture and socioenvironmental context.

According to Landrine and Klonoff, White Americans espouse a Western cultural view of health and illness. This view tends to focus on illness as person centered, and as an interpersonal condition caused by micro-level, natural, and etiological agents such as genes, viruses, bacteria, and stress. Illness or disease is seen as discrete and/or episodic. The implication of this is that treatment will be time limited. Furthermore, illness is conceptualized and treated without reference to God, community, nature, or the family. Landrine and Klonoff note that this view results in medical care that is discrete, segmented, and episodic in nature. This view also assumes that only experts are trained in the diagnosis and treatment of the disease.

In contrast to the more person-centered approach of Western culture regarding illness and disability, Landrine and Klonoff note that many non-Western groups, including some ethnic minority groups in the United States, view illness as long-term, fluid, and continuous manifestation of long-term and dynamic relationships within the family, community, or nature. The schemas of these individuals include macro-level, interpersonal, and supernatural causes as explanations for illness or disease. One implication of the belief that an illness does not originate within the person is that the individual may not comply with Western treatment or recommendations.

According to Landrine and Klonoff, cultures that support the non-Western worldview of health and illness provide several alternative explanations for the causes of illness. These explanations assume that illnesses are caused by (a) violations of interpersonal norms; (b) deviations from social roles and norms; (c) certain emotions such as jealousy and envy that may provoke disease; (d) violations of religious and moral norms; and (e) certain agents found in nature such as weather conditions and hot or cold foods.

In a review of explanations for illness, Murdock (1989) (cited in Landrine & Klonoff, 1992) found that theories about the causes of illness can be categorized into two major types: theories of natural causation and theories of supernatural causation. Theories of natural causation include viruses, infection, aging, accidents, homicides, and stress as the causes of illness. Theories of supernatural causation include causes such as mystical retribution (punishment by the gods for violating rules), animistic causation (soul loss or spirit aggression for violating rules), and magical causation (witchcraft, "evil eye"). In an examination of 189 different cultures, Murdock found that the beliefs of only four cultures included natural explanation for illness.

Some ethnic minority and cultural groups in the United States may also hold supernatural beliefs about the causes of illness. The beliefs that illness and disease are supernaturally caused have been documented among African Americans in the United States. The author is reminded of conversations with African Americans who held beliefs that certain persons have the power to put a hex or a spell causing illness on them or someone else. Such supernatural beliefs about the cause of illness and disease promote supernatural explanations for the treatment of illness and disease.

For example, within the African American community, there have been healers such as *root doctors* who were used to cure illness and disease. Root doctors used roots and herbs in treatments of physical, mental, and social conditions. Using the previous example, when a hex or spell was cast, it could only be broken by a root doctor. In some parts of the United States, the root doctors held positions of high status and prestige in the community. While root doctors are no longer prevalent within the African American community, there are some anecdotal accounts that they still exist, especially in certain areas of the South. It is interesting that many individuals from all ethnic groups are now using herbs and roots to maintain health and treat disease.

Other healers in the African American community provided nontraditional health care. Bailey (1990) provided an interesting history of the early evolution of folk health practitioners in one city in the United

States. Bailey studied patterns of health care use among Detroit African Americans from 1910 to 1939 and noted that a large percentage of African Americans consulted various folk health practitioners for several reasons. These included: (a) a need to cope with health problems within their own community and social environment; (b) a belief that folk health practitioners had some control over the forces that cause problems or abnormalities in the person's life; (c) less expensive cost of treatment; and (d) a need to be involved in the family's care, nurturing, and healing process. Bailey noted that folk health practitioners were adaptable and diverse in their abilities and specialized skills.

While faith healers are not unique to the African-American community, they have prospered here with their therapy of laying on of hands. These faith or spiritual healers, also known as spiritualists and Divine Healers, have played a prominent role within the treatment of African Americans with health and medical concerns. These healers, are believed to possess the power to cure disease. In an account of the prosperity of divine healers, Washington noted, "One of these healers started in business only a month ago, charging 50 cents a treatment. He has built up such a following that he is now charging from $2.00 to $25.00, according to the amount he thinks a patient will be able to pay. His office is always full of sick Blacks who get up early in the morning to be the first in line when his place of business opens" (Washington, cited in Bailey).

Within the African American community, the nonmedical healers fulfilled practical, as well as spiritual, functions. Given poor socioeconomic conditions and a history of racism, the health care system has not been accessible to all African Americans. The root doctor and other healers offered hope and faith that one would get better. These nontraditional healers lived within the community and were accessible and relatively inexpensive. Furthermore, the family was often acknowledged and/or involved in the treatment regimen. While faith healers and divine healers are not prevalent within the African American community today, there are still remnants of methods used by these individuals. This is evidenced by present-day testimonials, witnessing, and other expressions of spirituality and faith as a prerequisite to healing.

There is historical as well as theoretical support for the role of faith and spirituality in treatment. The power of faith and meditation has been documented since antiquity. If one has strong beliefs that one will recover and/or improve, this enhances the likelihood of improvement. This is akin to self-efficacy beliefs, which are discussed in chapter 8. The individual is more likely to have thoughts of and engage in behaviors to facilitate recovery and optimal functioning. The other beneficial aspect of faith is that it provides an adaptive coping strategy, so that a person is better able to deal with and accept the challenge and/or limitations of his/her health status, disability, or impairment.

Among African Americans, supernatural explanations may be given for the causes of disabling conditions. Toliver-Weddington (1990) writes that some African Americans show the same patterns of etiology of disabling conditions as can be found in Africa. For example, Nigerian mothers assumed that cleft palate was caused by evil spirits, that the spirits were angered by the mothers staying in the sun too long, or that the spirits for some were sent by others (Nwanze & Sowemino, 1987, cited in Toliver-Weddington, 1990). Nwanze & Sowemino noted that these beliefs are similar to those of some African Americans, who believed that a cleft lip can be caused when a pregnant woman is frightened by a rabbit, if she makes a mockery of someone with a similar problem, or is being punished for vanity.

In summary, the literature suggests that views of illness and disease are influenced by culture. Western conceptualizations of the etiology focus on disease and illness as person centered as opposed to non-Western cultures, in which views of illness and disease may be seen as caused by forces outside the individual. Some of the beliefs in more supernatural explanations for the cause of illness and disease are held among African Americans today, although to a lesser degree. These beliefs may be mediated by socioeconomic status and other demographic factors such as the region of the country where a person resides and age.

CULTURAL AND ETHNIC ISSUES IN ATTITUDES TOWARD PERSONS WITH DISABILITIES

One of the implications of a supernatural etiology for chronic illness and disability is that the individual and/or ancestors might have done something (consciously or unconsciously) to bring on the condition. Given this type of attribution for a disabling condition, one might expect less tolerance or more negative attitudes toward persons with disabilities among African Americans than among White Americans. An alternative explanation is that the person is not accountable for the illness or disability because this condition has occurred because of forces outside the individual's control. This interpretation should result in a more external attribution for illness or disability and more tolerant attitudes toward persons with disabilities.

In general, the literature suggests that persons with disabilities are stigmatized and more likely to be devalued as a group relative to persons without disabilities (Esses & Beaufoy, 1994; Wright, 1960; Yuker, 1994). The level of stigmatization and intolerance seems to be mediated by ethnicity. The literature suggests that there is more acceptance and positive attitudes toward people with disabilities among African Americans than Caucasians (Grand & Strohmer, 1983). In a study of attitudes toward persons with disabilities, using college students as subjects, Grand and

Strohmer (1983) found that African Americans had more positive attitudes than White Americans. The authors speculated that this difference might be in part due to perceived similarity of stigmatization and minority group status among African Americans and persons with disabilities.

Another explanation for more favorable attitudes among African Americans is related to core African values that African Americans may possess. Among African Americans, interpersonal and spiritual relationships take precedence over materialistic and achievement-related orientations. Within this context, the relationship with another person is of highest value, regardless of whether the person has a disability that might limit (at least in the perceiver's eyes) the ability to achieve and produce in a materialistic sense (Myers, 1988).

Attitudes toward self affect functioning within every domain, (i.e., work, family, community). For persons with disabilities, acceptance of self and one's disability are key to healthy, adaptive functioning. In order to function effectively, there must be positive regard for oneself as a member of a community of persons with disabilities. There must also be acceptance of oneself as an African American.

Acceptance of disability is favorable to the extent that a person (a) is able to value things other than those that are in direct conflict with his or her disability; (b) is able to deemphasize aspects of physical ability and appearance that contradict his or her disabled situation; (c) does not feel handicapped by the disability other than beyond the actual impairment limitations; and (d) does not compare himself or herself to others in terms of areas of limitations but emphasizes his or her own assets and abilities (Wright, 1960).

In a study of 170 African Americans with disabilities, Belgrave (1991) investigated the influence of several psychological and sociological variables on acceptance of disability. The results of this study indicated that perception of disability severity, social support, and self-esteem were significant contributors to adjustment to disability. Thus, feeling good about oneself and having support from family and friends were important to adjustment for these African Americans. Similarly, the perception that the disability was not severe was associated with more favorable acceptance. To the extent that persons with disabilities can engage in activities and receive affirmations that enhance feelings of self-worth, have good support from family and friends, and do not perceive that they are limited by the disabling condition will there be positive acceptance of self.

AFRICENTRIC FRAMEWORK

Acceptance of self also involves acceptance of one's history and culture. African Americans share a history based on African culture and a legacy of slavery and oppression in the United States. Much of African American behavior can be traced to African culture and values modified by experiences in America (Hale-Benson, 1986). Several scholars have written on the Africentric worldview or beliefs (Akbar, 1979; Asante, 1988; Azibo, 1989, 1996; Baldwin, 1981, 1990; Myers, 1988; Nobles, 1986, 1990; Phillips, 1990). This Africentric worldview provides a useful framework for understanding attitudes and behaviors among persons of African descent. Similarly, this Africentric framework is useful for providing a framework in which to understand the influence of culture on the experiencing of chronic illness and disability among African Americans.

An Africentric worldview is values, beliefs, and ways of behavior that characterize people of African descent. While there is a great degree of diversity among African Americans, this worldview is assumed to be prescribed to in varying degrees by a substantial number of African Americans in the United States.

Many African American scholars maintain that this worldview is adaptive and necessary for optimal functioning for African Americans (Azibo, 1989, 1996; Myers, 1988; Nobles, 1986). In writing on African American personality, Azibo (1989) suggests that deviation from core Africentric values may lead to pathology among African Americans.

The assumption made here is that adherence to Africentric values can facilitate functioning and positive outcomes among African Americans with disabilities. Atkins (1988) also emphasizes this point. According to her, it is important to have a philosophy wherein cultural values are considered assets rather than deficits. She writes, "asset orientation reflects a belief that positive outcomes originate from shaping strengths and failure results from a concentration on limitations, fears, and negatives" (p. 45).

Randolph and Banks (1993) summarized nine dimensions or qualities of the African worldview that have been articulated by several African American scholars, including Naim Akbar, Daudi Azibo, Joseph Baldwin, Wade Boykins, Asa Hilliard, Linda J. Myers, Edwin Nichols, and Wade Nobles among others. They include the following:

1. *Spirituality*. This is the acknowledgment that there is a presence or force greater than oneself. There is a relationship with God or some other supernatural being. This orientation emphasizes the spiritual over the material. Spirituality provides the foundation for meaning and direction to one's life and permeates every aspect of being. Spirituality is often (but not always) manifested by worship, prayers, and other rituals that are symbolic and strengthen one's spiritual connection. A spiritual basis provides a foundation or reason for being.

2. *Interpersonal orientation/communalism.* Interrelatedness and connection to others characterize this orientation. Interpersonal and affiliative relationships may be valued over materialistic or production-oriented activities. This worldview emphasizes a belief in the importance of the group over the individual and cooperation rather than competition. The self is viewed as part of a collective phenomenon. The axiom "I am because we are" typifies this dimension. An interpersonal communal orientation recognizes the value of the person irrespective of his or her physical condition and production of materialistic things.
3. *Harmony.* This is the belief that all aspects of one's life must be integrated. All dimensions of one's being—physical, spiritual, emotional, vocational—are connected. Persons holding this belief believe that optimal functioning is not possible unless all aspects of one's life are in balance. This orientation would support the belief that one's disability and physical self are a part of who one is. This representation should encourage favorable self-acceptance.
4. *Time as a social phenomenon.* This dimension relates to the previous one in that all things flow into one another, and events are not discrete and unconnected. The clock or calendar does not dictate when something begins or ends. The occurrence of events is dictated by the will of the people, not by the clock. This is exemplified by the saying "the party starts when the people arrive."
5. *Affect sensitivity to emotional cues (synthesis of the verbal and nonverbal).* This involves sensitivity to the feelings and the emotional needs of others. The expression and perception of feelings is seen in nonverbal as well as verbal behavior. Emotions and feelings are expressed verbally and nonverbally, and one is in tune with how others feel.
6. *Expressive communication/orality.* Oral expression is a preferred means of communication. Information transmitted orally carries equal weight to that which is written. Communication may not be direct (or it may); it will be expressive and fluid. Art, dance, speech, music, and body movements and position may be used to convey thoughts and ideas. This orientation has implication for communicating with an African American with a disability. Here, a personal conversation regarding adherence instructions may be more effective than an impersonal written list of instructions.
7. *Rhythmic movement and stylistic expressiveness.* This orientation recognizes the uniqueness of each person's flair, style, and man-

ner of expression. Spontaneity and improvisation are emphasized to the extent that it facilitates group goals. This unique manner of expression can be seen in the African American's way of walking, dressing, and communicating with others.

8. *Multidimensional perception/verve (multimodal perception and learning).* Learning preferences are multidimensional and include visual, auditory, tactile, and motor channels simultaneously. There is a preference for a variety of stimuli. This orientation would support the notion that a variety of methods might be necessary for encouraging preventive and treatment adherence.
9. *Negativity to positivity.* This orientation reflects the ability to turn a bad situation into a positive one; to see something good derived from something bad. The positivity orientation will have a favorable influence on acceptance of disability and potentially aversive conditions. The author is reminded of conversations with persons who had stressful situations thrust upon them. Many have taken these situations and found something positive.

While a great deal of diversity exists among African Americans, these values exist more or less among persons of African descent throughout the diaspora. The transmission of these Africentric values modified by experiences in America have shaped the values, behaviors, and beliefs among African Americans today. A history of slavery, racism, and oppression contributed to the evolution of systems that met the needs of African Americans. One such system is the extended African American family. African American extended kin networks have been a central structure in African and African American family life (Martin & Martin, 1978) and crucial to the survival and adaptation of African Americans in this country (Wilson, 1989).

McAdoo (1981) described the extended family as a "help network" in which there is reciprocal obligation to help relatives who may be biological or nonbiological. This network provides not only a bond and an emotional connection, but economical and financial support as well. Members of the family who are able are expected to help the less able. Members of the family who do not have jobs are expected to help in other ways (i.e., baby-sit for those who do go to work). The African American family network is further characterized by frequent contact whereby close relationships are developed with cousins and other relatives. Relationships may also be developed with fictive kin, those individuals who are treated as if they are members of the family although they are not biologically related or related through marriage. In some cases, these relatives may live in the same house or in close proximity to one another. It can be seen that this interdependence and connection among families is an extension of Africentric values, which emphasize interpersonal, communal, and affiliative relationships. The extended kin reciprocity has also been reinforced by a legacy of oppression which dictated that African Americans look out for and help one another.

Respect for elders is another characteristic of African American families that originated from Africa. Children are responsible for the care and welfare of their parents and older relatives are expected to spend their last years in the homes of relatives rather than in nursing homes (Toliver-Weddington, 1990). This same respect and sharing of responsibilities may also be evidenced among African Americans who may assist in caring for persons who are less able to physically or mentally take care of themselves.

THE IMPACT OF CULTURE AND AFRICENTRIC VALUES ON FUNCTIONING OF PERSONS WITH CHRONIC ILLNESSES AND DISABILITIES

The cultural values and Africentric worldview impact the experiences of all African Americans to a certain degree. They can also both facilitate and impede adaptive functioning among African Americans with chronic illnesses and disabilities.

Extended Family Network

The extended family can be an asset for a person with a disability who may need support in a number of areas. For example, some individuals with disabilities may be isolated and have limited participation in everyday activities outside the home. Within African American extended families, however, there may be less isolation because of ties to persons within and outside the immediate family. The presence of the extended family among African Americans with disabilities was seen in a study by Belgrave, Davis, & Vadja, 1994. In a study of providers of social support for African Americans with disabilities, they found that African Americans listed more kin than White Americans although there was no difference between the two groups in the number of immediate family members listed. The findings from this study suggest that the networks of African Americans with disabilities are more likely to include more significant others outside the immediate family. This extended family may provide emotional support and reassurance, as well as material support (i.e., help with transportation, baby-sitting, etc.). Extended family also provides an additional buffer for dealing with stress or problems within the household. The extended family is likely to live in the community and be in frequent contact with the family.

An understanding of who is in the extended family and what functions these individuals serve may help us understand why and how medical and rehabilitation services are accessed. For example, when working with a consumer, it may be helpful to know who will assist the individual in going to his or her appointment or who will provide transportation.

The importance of the extended family in employment outcomes of African Americans with disabilities was seen in a study by Walker et al. (1995). In this study, Walker et al. examined how support from various sources related to employment beliefs. These beliefs were expected to contribute to whether or not people found a job. Using a mostly African American sample, the authors found that support from family was related to one's beliefs that he or she would secure employment. Support from professionals was not related to employment beliefs. This finding provides support for the involvement of family in rehabilitation and medical activities for African Americans.

Communal and Group Orientation

Having a communal and group orientation may be adaptive among African Americans with disabilities for several reasons. One, achievement of the individual is subordinate to the achievement of the group. Thus, an individual is respected because he or she is a member of a group rather than for his or her individual achievements. As noted, success is not necessarily defined by the acquisition of material goods, education, or status, but by the viability of the family and the group. Under conditions whereby a person is not able to achieve material success because of a disability or impairment, one's status within the community would not diminish.

An Africentric worldview assumes that a communal or group approach will be useful when working with African Americans with disabilities. In our work, we have found this to be true. In groups we have run, goals of group members are defined by the group and the major task of the group is for members to help each other. For example, when one member of the group found employment, all members of the group took credit for this success. Conversely, when members of the group failed to find work, all members were disappointed.

Spirituality

Belief in a power or force greater than oneself is very comforting to those undergoing stress and turmoil. Spirituality provides a framework for that which is incomprehensible. It also provides hope and faith for a better life. Turning one's life over to God or a higher power facilitates acceptance of adversity and hard times because there is the acknowledgment that there is a purpose and a reason to all things.

There has been some research that has shown that spirituality is an adaptive coping response for African Americans. Cheung and Snowden (1990) have identified religion, prayer, and spirituality as key ways of coping among African Americans. According to Cheung and Snowden, Blacks use prayer more than Whites as a response to problems. In their study on stress and coping among African Americans, Neighbors, Jackson, Bowman, and Gurin (1983) confirmed the extensive use of prayer and noted that as the seriousness of the problems increased, so did the number of African Americans who felt that prayer helped them the most.

Being part of a spiritual and religious network also serves an additional practical function of increasing the number of persons in the network. Ministers, deacons, and other church members fulfill many of the support functions of the extended families and in effect become members of the extended family.

Negativity to Positivity

This worldview can be quite adaptive in getting persons through tough times. It is related to spirituality, in that good is seen as coming from something bad. I found in interviews with African American women who were HIV positive that frequently these women mentioned that the positive HIV diagnosis helped to turn their lives around, made them stop and reassess their priorities, and put them in touch with God and their faith. In other words, they had turned a negative into a positive.

Similarly, when an African American or a member of his or her family acquires a chronic illness or disabling condition, there may be a positive reinterpretation of this event. In a study of parents with children with disabilities, Walker and Belgrave (1995) found that African American parents were likely to report the use of positive reinterpretation as a coping strategy. In interviews with these parents several reported positive outcomes. Parents, for example, reported that they became stronger, that the experience had strengthened their faith, and that the experience had made them grow stronger as a family.

Harmony

As noted, symptoms and functional limitations resulting from a disability or chronic illness are not seen as discrete, something that can be treated separately from other aspects of the individual's life. When one sync is out of order, everything is out of order. The implication for treatment is that the physical, spiritual, and social aspects of the individual have to be considered when medical and rehabilitative services are provided.

SUMMARY

The culture of African Americans influences their perception of and adaptation to chronic illness and disability. Africentric values are derived from African culture and are shaped by American socialization. Africentric values include spirituality, communalism, harmony, time as a social phenomenon, affect and sensitivity, orality, rhythmic movement, multidimensional perception, extended family, and respect for elders.

African Americans may have schemas about disability and chronic illness that are more consistent with a non-Western conceptualization than a Western conceptualization. Chronic illness and disability are not likely to be seen and treated as concrete, episodic events but as events that are much more integrated within other aspects of the individual's life and within his or her social group. Cultural values, worldview, and beliefs must be taken into consideration when conducting research and developing programs for African Americans with chronic illnesses and disabilities.

PART II

Adaptive Functioning

4

Factors Contributing to Employment Success Among African Americans with Disabilities

African Americans with chronic illnesses and disabilities face a formidable challenge in the employment arena. Only 22% of working-age (persons aged 16 to 64) African Americans with disabilities are in the labor force (i.e., employed or seeking employment), and only 16% are actually working (Bowe, 1985, 1991; Alston & Mngadi, 1992). This leaves the vast majority not working or seeking work. While some persons cannot work because of the limitations of a chronic illness or disability, most want to work and in fact have the ability to work productively.

Factors that facilitate (or impede) employment are an important area of investigation and are the scope of this chapter. Work (or the lack of it) affects the quality of life across several dimensions. In this country, work is tied to self-worth, self-esteem, and feelings of accomplishment. Work impacts interpersonal and social relationships within the home and the community. Perhaps most importantly, having a job determines whether or not one has a basic standard of living with adequate food, shelter, and medical care. For African Americans, people with disabili-

The author would like to thank Dr. Sylvia Walker at the Howard University Research & Training Center for Access to Rehabilitation and Economic Opportunity for her support of this research. The research was funded by the National Institute of Disability and Rehabilitation Research in a grant to Howard University (Dr. Sylvia Walker, Principal Investigator).

ties, and other oppressed groups, employment is especially important. Work is a mechanism for gaining equity and control in one's life. Because of the central role that employment plays, this chapter is devoted to a better understanding of factors that contribute to employment success. Chapters 7 and 8 discuss strategies I have used with colleagues to improve employability among African Americans with disabilities.

In this chapter, research conducted by the author and colleagues on factors related to employment success among African Americans with disabilities is presented. This research was aimed at identifying factors that account for successful employment among African Americans with disabilities and chronic illnesses.

EARLIER RESEARCH ON EMPLOYMENT OUTCOMES

Two earlier studies are relevant to the research discussed in this chapter and are briefly reviewed. The findings from these studies pointed to several demographic, psychological, and sociological factors associated with employment among African Americans with disabilities (Belgrave & Walker, 1991a & b; Wilson, 1988).

Wilson (1988) conducted a qualitative study on critical factors in the employment success of African Americans with disabilities. He used a case study methodology to identify critical factors in the lives of successfully employed African Americans with disabilities.

Wilson identified seven successful African Americans. Data on these individuals were gathered from various publications and public source materials. Two of the individuals were born with impairments, two acquired disabilities during their teen years, and the other three acquired a disability in their adult years after being successfully employed as able-bodied persons. Three were impaired by blindness, one by dwarfism and the absence of hands and arms, one by amputations of both arms above the elbow, one by multiple sclerosis, and one by quadriplegia. The individuals were successfully employed as an executive director of a community program, a manager of a women's project, a rehabilitation administrator, a minister, a social worker, a community activist, and a director of community relations.

Extensive information was gathered and reviewed on these individuals. Key factors operative across all individuals are summarized below:

a. Career path.—Five of these individuals had a stable career path; the other two had a varied employment path but were successful in their careers.

b. Family background.—Six of the individuals came from family backgrounds that were intact. All of these individuals had the presence of at least one strong, highly moral parent. The work ethic was also present among families.

c. Self-concept or confidence.—All individuals were goal directed and had confidence in their abilities to achieve.
d. Religion or spirituality.—The majority used religion or spirituality as an orienting theme in their lives.
e. Realistic self-appraisal.—The disability experiences required that these individuals face reality and engage in adaptive problem-solving solutions. These individuals had good coping mechanisms for dealing with frustration. All had potential mobility or transportation problems but learned how to meet their needs for getting around.
f. Understands and copes effectively with devaluation.—These individuals did not focus on racism or handicapism and when it occurred knew how to deal with it.
g. Preference for long-term goals.—These individuals had a preference for long-term goals that provided them with tenacity as they moved through the rehabilitation process.
h. Availability of strong support.—These individuals all needed, accepted, and benefited from support. Support was in the form of positive regard and acceptance, information, treatment, and opportunities for development and employment.
i. Demonstrated leadership.—All persons were leaders in some aspect and were recognized for this leadership.
j. Demonstrated community service.—All individuals provided services to various communities.
k. Sharing of knowledge.—All individuals shared their special knowledge and expertise with others.

Wilson's research made an important contribution to understanding employment issues because it demonstrated that African Americans with disabilities could be very successful. Moreover, Wilson focused on identifying strengths rather than deficits. And by including only successful subjects in the case study, his research focused on success rather than failure. However, the findings from this study are limited because of the methodology. Only seven persons were selected for the case study. Moreover, since Wilson relied upon published documents and public information on these persons, these individuals would probably be considered noteworthy and exceptional. There are thousands of African Americans with disabilities and chronic illnesses who are productive at work, earn a decent living, and contribute to society. These ordinary individuals would not be in the public eye. What factors motivate successful employment among these individuals?

Belgrave and Walker (1991a & b) conducted a study on predictors of employment status among African Americans with disabilities. They were interested in identifying psychological and demographic factors that were related to whether or not a person was employed. Seven variables were tested: social support, self-esteem, locus of control, perception of disability severity, acceptance of disability, availability of transportation, and education.

Participants in the Belgrave and Walker study were 75 African Americans with disabilities who ranged in age from 21 to 45. Disabilities included vision and hearing impairments, orthopedic impairments, kidney failure, cardiovascular and respiratory impairments, and spinal cord injury. Data were collected from participants through a questionnaire or interview that contained measures of the variables of interest. Thirty-two percent were employed, and 68% were not employed.

A discriminate analysis was conducted to determine which variables significantly discriminated between those who were employed and unemployed. The results of this analysis revealed that two variables significantly discriminated the employed from the not-employed group. These variables were transportation source and social support. Employed respondents were more likely to own or have access to cars or other privately owned vehicles and use these for transportation. Unemployed respondents were more likely to use public transportation such as bus or train as their primary mode of transportation. The relationship between employment and vehicle ownership is circular. Employed persons are more likely than unemployed persons to be able to afford a vehicle, and having a vehicle probably facilitates finding and keeping a job.

The perception of the availability of social support was also a significant discriminator between those who were employed and unemployed. Employed persons were more likely than nonemployed persons to feel that social support was available when needed.

The research by Wilson (1988) and Belgrave and Walker (1991a & b) provided a preliminary understanding of factors that may contribute to whether or not African Americans with disabilities are employed. However, these studies were limited in terms of methodology and the conceptualization of the predictor and the outcome variables. As noted, in the Wilson study only individuals who were successfully employed and notable in their field were included. In the Belgrave and Walker study, the outcome variable of employment status (i.e., whether or not the individual was working) was somewhat limited and did not consider other indicators of employment success such as attitudes toward employment. Attitudes toward work are important outcome variables in their own right. Positive attitudes toward employment are likely to increase efforts to find employment if unemployed and motivate the individual to remain employed. Among African Americans with disabilities, the vast majority are unemployed. Therefore, a first step may be to increase their attitudes regarding the value of work and their beliefs that they can find and maintain work. These outcomes were the focus of the intervention programs described in chapters 7 and 8.

A study on factors related to employment success among African Americans with disabilities was conducted to address some of the concerns of the previous studies. Employment success was conceptualized more comprehensively than in the other studies and two indicators of employment success were used. One, employment status, (i.e., whether or not the individual was actually employed) was an outcome that was similar to the one used in the previous study (Belgrave & Walker, 1991a & b). Two, "attitudes toward employment" was added as an additional outcome variable. Favorable work attitudes are likely to motivate the employed to continue working and motivate the unemployed to be persistent in their employment search. Another improvement in this study was in the conceptualization of the predictor variables. The selection of predictor variables in the Belgrave and Walker (1991a & b) study was not based on any one theoretical model, but a hodgepodge of factors hypothesized to affect employment based on a review of the literature. In this study the authors wanted to test whether one theoretical model could parsimoniously account for employment success.

A MODEL OF RISK AND RESISTANCE FACTORS AS PREDICTORS OF VOCATIONAL OUTCOMES

We selected a model that we felt was flexible enough to account for adaptive functioning in the employment domain for our target population of African Americans with disabilities. Wallander and colleagues' risk and resistance model seemed appropriate and was adapted for the study (Wallander & Varni, 1989; Wallander, Feldman & Varni, 1989; Wallander et al., 1989). Wallander and colleagues' model accounts for differential levels of psychosocial adjustment in children with disabilities (Varni, Wilcox, & Hanson, 1988). While the model has been used in studies with chronically ill and disabled children, it seemed useful for conceptualizing outcomes among African Americans with disabilities.

According to the model, behavioral adjustment to a disability or chronic illness can be accounted for by two general sets of factors—risk factors and resistance factors. Risk factors can be grouped into three categories as follows: (a) disease and disability parameters (i.e., disability severity, level of cognitive functioning, type of disability); (b) level of functional independence (e.g., ability to function in activities of daily living); and (c) psychosocial stressors (i.e., major life events, daily stressors, etc.).

Resistance factors are those that moderate (or resist) the impact of stress and the disability and include (a) intrapersonal factors (e.g., perceived competence, self-esteem, motivation); (b) socioecological factors (i.e., social support, family environment); and (c) stress processing factors (i.e., coping strategies, beliefs).

Tests of the model have shown a much stronger impact of resistance factors on adjustment than risk factors (Wallander et al., 1989). That is, factors such as coping style of parents, social support, and family environment seem to explain behavioral adjustment much better than risk factors such as type of and severity of disability (Varni, Wilcox, & Hanson, 1988; Varni, Setoguchi, Rappaport, & Talbot 1992; Wallander et al., 1989).

The three resistance factors and one risk factor (severity of disability) were included in this study. Self-esteem was selected as an intrapersonal resistance factor. Prior research had demonstrated self-esteem to be associated with favorable disability outcomes (Belgrave, 1991; Wilson, 1988). Social support was selected as the socioecological resistance variable. There is extensive evidence of the facilitative role that social support plays in enhancing outcomes of African Americans with disabilities (see chapter 5). A stress-processing variable for persons with a disability is their beliefs about what it means to have a disability. Beliefs that a disability is not limiting and that persons with disabilities can achieve desired goals should facilitate adaptive functioning.

Other factors, such as demographic variables, that might affect employment success (e.g., age, education, marital status, living situation), rehabilitation service utilization, and vocational history variables (e.g., usual occupation, work history, and perceived ability to work) were also included in the model.

The methodology used to conduct the study is discussed in the next section followed by the results and a summary of the results and implications.

Method

Participants. The sample consisted of 186 African Americans with disabilities whose age ranged from 20 to 64. Respondents were clients of or affiliated with rehabilitation facilities, agencies, and hospitals. These facilities were selected because they were in cities where African Americans comprise a substantial percentage of the population. These agencies and facilities were Harlem Hospital, New York, New York; Michigan Department of Rehabilitation, Detroit, Michigan; California Department of Rehabilitation, Los Angeles, California; Georgia Department of Rehabilitation, Atlanta, Georgia; Atlanta Independent Living Center, Atlanta, Georgia; and Rehabilitation Services Agency, Washington, DC. Respondents were randomly selected from a list of clients at each agency.

Respondents reported a variety of disabling conditions. One hundred fourteen had a physical disability, 9 had a cognitive disability, 35 had an emotional disability, and 17 had a sensory disability. The type of disability was not identified for 11 subjects.

Procedures. Contact persons at each site were identified by the Howard University Research and Training Center on Disability (R&T Center) and asked to participate in the study. In most cases, these organizations had been involved in earlier studies with the R&T Center. Contact persons at each of the sites were responsible for identifying and recruiting respondents. As noted, all respondents had some affiliation with the participating site (e.g., as a client, resident, patient, etc.). Data were collected in 1991.

The questionnaire was administered by a trained interviewer, usually a rehabilitation specialist, at each site. Administration time took about an hour. Respondents were given a small stipend upon completion of the interview.

Measures. The predictor variables were attitudes toward disability, social support, and self-esteem. Demographic, vocational, medical, and rehabilitation variables were also included as predictor variables. The dependent (outcome) variables were employment and attitudes toward employment.

The structured interview protocol developed by Walker and Asbury (1993) was used to obtain measures. This protocol contained several measures to comprehensively assess respondents' attitudes, beliefs, and behaviors along several dimensions related to rehabilitation utilization and employment (Walker & Asbury, 1993). Measures relevant to this study are reviewed below.

Measures of Predictor Variables. The 10-item Rosenberg (1965) self-esteem scale was used to measure self-esteem. Respondents responded to statements about themselves on a 1 (strongly agree) to a 7 (strongly disagree) scale. This scale has been used in numerous studies and has acceptable reliability and validity.

The social support scale measured two types of social support—emotional and tangible (material) as well as combined social support (Walker & Asbury, 1993). The emotional scale was composed of 10 items, and the tangible support scale was comprised of nine items. Respondents responded to statements on a 1 (strongly agree) to a 7 (strongly disagree) scale.

Attitudes toward disability were assessed by an 18-item scale (Walker & Asbury, 1993). These items were written to assess the respondent's perception of his/her disability, including the extent to which the disability is perceived both positively and negatively. Examples of scale items are: (1) My disability prevents me from doing just about everything I really want to do and from becoming the kind of person I want to be and (2) I feel satisfied with my abilities, and my disability doesn't bother me too much. Participants responded to statements describing their attitudes toward their disability on a 1 (strongly agree) to a 7 (strongly disagree) scale.

Demographic variables were assessed by asking respondents their age, level of education, and marital status. Rehabilitation service utilization was assessed by asking respondents whether or not they were currently receiving or had received rehabilitation services over the past year. Vocational variables were assessed with the following questions: (1) What is your usual occupation? (2) Did you work prior to becoming disabled? (3) Do you have the capacity to do the same type of work? (4) Do you want to work?

Measures of Dependent Variables. Employment status was derived from respondents' response to the following question: Which of the following best describes your employment status: (a) employed, (b) unemployment and not looking for work, (c) not employed but looking for work, (d) laid off temporarily, and (e) retired. Categories b, c, and d were combined to comprise the not-employed category. Respondents who were retired were not included in analyses.

Attitude toward work was assessed by an attitude toward employment scale (Walker & Asbury, 1993). This scale consists of eight items, which assess the extent to which a person values employment and feels that employment is important. This scale ranged from 1 (strongly agree) to 6 (strongly disagree). An example of an item from the scale is "I feel that productive work is an essential part of living a full life."

Results

Descriptive Statistics on Sample. Descriptive statistics on the sample are shown in Table 4.1. The age ranged from 20 to 64 with a mean age of 39.7. The sample had slightly more males than females. The majority were not married and had no children. About 30% lived alone; the remainder lived with a spouse, child, parent, or another person. The majority of the respondents had at least a high school or higher level of education. Employment income was very low, with 37% of the sample reporting income derived from employment as under $2,000, 25% reporting income from employment between $2,000 and $10,000, and 37% reporting income from employment above $10,000. Note that these figures would probably be higher in 1998.

Descriptive Statistics on Vocational and Rehabilitation Variables. Descriptive statistics on vocational variables are shown in Table 4.2. Forty-two percent of the sample were employed, and 57.6% were not employed. About 10% had never been employed. The majority of respondents reported their usual occupation as blue-collar, followed by clerical

Table 4.1
Descriptive Statistics on Sample (N = 186)

Age		
	Mean	39.7
	Range	20-64
	S.D.	12.5
		%
Sex		
	Female	43.2
	Male	56.8
Marital status		
	Single	58.5
	Married	41.5
Living situation		
	Live alone	30.1
	With spouse/child	19.9
	With parent(s)	22.6
	Other	27.4
Education		
	< H.S.	27.4
	H.S.	44.8
	> H.S.	27.9
Children		
	None	52.4
	One or more	47.5
Income from employment		
	< $2,000	37.7
	$2,000 -10,000	25.4
	> $10,000	37.0

and professional. The majority thought that they were capable of doing the same type of work they had done before becoming disabled. Slightly more had worked (than not worked) prior to becoming disabled (54.4% versus 45.5%). A large majority, 77.8%, reported that they had the ability to work, and an overwhelming majority, 93.6%, reported a desire to work.

Respondents in this sample had very favorable attitudes toward employment. The average score was 5.1 out of a high possible score of 6.

Descriptive statistics on rehabilitation variables are in Table 4.2. The majority, 59.6%, were not currently receiving rehabilitation services, although a majority, 66.4%, had received such services in the past.

The interviewer provided an assessment of his or her perception of the severity of the respondent's disability on a scale that ranged from 1 (minimally disabled) to 7 (very severely disabled). The average rating

Table 4.2
Descriptive Statistics on Vocational, Medical, and Rehabilitation Variables

		%
Employment*		
	Employed	42.4
	Not employed	57.6
Usual Occupation		
	Never employed	9.8
	Blue collar	37.6
	Clerical	21.0
	Professional	19.3
	Other	12.2
If unemployed, perceived ability to work		
	Yes	77.8
	No	22.2
Desire to work		
	Yes	93.6
	No	6.4
Worked prior to disability		
	Yes	54.5
	No	45.5
Capacity to do same type of work		
	Yes	58.5
	No	41.5
Interviewer's assessment of probability of employment		
	Poor	30.7
	Fair	40.2
	Good	29.1

		%
Number of times hospitalized within past 2 years		
	None	61.5
	One or more	38.5
Number of times seen in emergency room within past 2 years		
	None	51.1
	One or more	48.9
Currently receiving rehabilitation services		
	Yes	40.6
	No	59.6
Received rehabilitation services in past		
	Yes	66.4
	No	33.6

Interviewer's assessment of disability severity	
Mean	3.1
Range	1-7
S.D.	1.5
Attitude toward employment	
Mean	5.1
Range	1-6
S.D.	.95

*Participants who were retired were not included.

was 3.1, suggesting a moderate rating of disability severity for these respondents.

Bivariate Analyses. Several bivariate analyses were computed to assess the relationships between predictor variables and dependent variables. The two dependent variables, employment status and attitudes toward employment, were significantly related to each other ($p < .05$). Persons not employed reported a less favorable attitude toward employment than did persons who were employed.

Variables Significantly Related to Employment Status. Variables significantly related to employment status are shown in Table 4.3. Only variables that were significant or marginally significant are included.

Respondents who were employed were rated as less severely disabled by the interviewer than respondents who were not employed. The mean ratings were 2.8 for the employed respondents and 3.3 for the unemployed respondents. This difference was marginally significant ($p < .07$).

Several vocational variables were significantly related to employment status. A higher percentage of the employed respondents reported their usual occupation as professional (22.9%) and blue-collar (41.4%), compared to the unemployed group. Only 15.8% of the unemployed respondents reported their usual occupation as professional, and only 32.6% reported their usual occupation as blue-collar.

Employed respondents compared to those not employed were also more likely to report that they were capable of performing their usual type of work. Employed respondents, compared to unemployed respondents, were more likely to perceive that they had the ability to work; 92.9% of the employed respondents versus 75.9% of the unemployed respondents felt they had the ability to work.

All three of the resistance variables were associated with employment status. The employed group scored significantly higher on the self-esteem measure than the not-employed group (mean = 5.2 versus 4.8). Similarly, the employed group had significantly more favorable beliefs about disability (mean = 4.7) than the not-employed group (mean = 4.4). Finally, the employed group reported receiving more emotional support (mean = 4.7) than the not employed group (mean = 4.4). This last difference was only marginally significant.

Variables Significantly Related to Attitudes Towards Employment. Gender and education were significantly correlated with attitudes toward employment. Men had more favorable attitudes toward employment than women. Higher levels of education were associated with more favorable attitudes toward employment.

The interviewer's assessment of the severity of the disability correlated negatively with attitudes toward employment. The more severe the interviewer rated the disability, the less favorable was the participant's

Table 4.3
Variables Significantly Related to Vocational Success and Probability Level

	Employment Status	Attitudes Toward Employment
Demographic variables		
Gender	-	.05
Education	-	.05
Medical variables		
Interviewer's assessment of disability severity	.07	.01
Vocational variables		
Usual occupation	.05	.05
Capacity to do same type of work	.002	-
Perceived ability to work	.05	-
Psychosocial Variables		
Self-esteem	.008	.08
Attitude toward disability	.009	.01
Perceived emotional support	.09	.01
Perceived material support	-	.01
Combined social support	-	.01

attitude toward employment. Participants whose usual occupations were clerical, blue-collar, and professional had more favorable attitudes than those who had never been employed.

All of the resistance factors correlated with attitudes toward work. High self-esteem was associated with more favorable attitudes. A more favorable perception of one's disability was correlated with more favorable employment attitudes. High levels of emotional and tangible support correlated with more favorable attitudes toward employment.

Multivariate Analyses with Predictor and Dependent Variables. Multivariate analyses were computed in order to determine the unique contribution of each of the predictor variables and the total amount of variance accounted for in the two dependent variables. Only variables that were significant in the bivariate analyses were included in the multivariate analyses. Variables that were categorical were coded into dichotomous variables.

A discriminant analysis was computed to determine which variables discriminated between those respondents who were employed and those respondents who were not employed (see Table 4.4). A significant canonical correlation ($p < .05$) accounted for 18% of the variance in employment status. Three of the predictor variables were significant. They were in order of influence (a) attitudes about the disability ($p < .03$); (b)

Table 4.4
Variables That Significantly Discriminated Between Employed and Nonemployed Group

Variable	Significance Level
Attitude toward disability	.01
Self-esteem	.01
Perceived capability to work	.01
Canonical correlation = .42	

self-esteem ($p < .01$); and (c) perceived capability to perform the same type of work ($p < .03$).

A stepwise multiple regression procedure was computed to determine which variables significantly explained attitudes toward employment (see Table 4.5). Nineteen percent of the variance in attitudes toward employment was accounted for ($p < .0001$). The three variables that were significant in order of influence were attitude toward disability ($p < .01$), disability severity ($p < .002$), and self-esteem ($p < .05$).

Summary and Implications of Study on Vocational Outcomes

The purpose of this study was to identify factors that related to employment success among African Americans with disabilities. A secondary purpose was to apply a model of risk and resistance factors to explaining employment outcomes.

Some of the findings from the descriptive statistics are noteworthy. The sample of African Americans had much higher employment rates than that found in the general population of African Americans with disabilities (i.e., 42% were employed). The overwhelming majority (94%) of the participants in this study reported a desire to work. Moreover, a large percentage, 78%, felt they had the ability to work. These findings suggest that work is valued in this population. Efforts to increase employability should be encouraged.

The findings from this study revealed several factors that relate to employment attitudes and behaviors. Disability severity was correlated with both measures. Respondents whose disabilities were rated as more severe had less successful employment outcomes. This finding is not surprising and supports the model of disability severity as a risk factor for adjustment.

Perceived capability to do the same type of work and perceived ability to work were significantly related to employment status. Participants who felt that they could continue to do the same type of work they had

Table 4.5
Variables That Significantly Predicted Attitudes Toward Employment

Variable	Significance Level
Disability severity	.003
Attitudes toward disability	.02
Self-esteem	.05

$R = .43$
$R^2 = .19$

done before becoming disabled were more likely to be employed and to have favorable work attitudes. Similarly participants who felt they had the ability to work were more likely to be employed. Persons whose usual occupation were blue-collar and professional were more likely to be employed than those whose occupations were not.

All three psychosocial variables related to employment status and attitudes toward employment in bivariate analysis. These findings are consistent with previous research by the author and others.

Multivariate Analyses. The multivariate analyses allowed us to assess the unique contribution of the resistance and risk factors on the two vocational variables. For the employment status measure, attitudes toward the disability, self-esteem, and perceived capability to do the same type of work were significant factors. For the attitudes toward employment measure, severity of disability, attitudes toward the disability, and self-esteem were significant predictors.

Self-esteem appears to have an important influence on vocational success. The importance of self-esteem as it relates to vocational success is highlighted by the fact that it was a significant predictor for both of the employment measures and was significant in both bivariate and multivariate analyses.

Attitudes toward disability were also an influential variable. They were also a significant predictor in both the multivariate and bivariate analyses. This is not surprising; self-esteem and attitude toward disability are closely related. Disabled persons who feel positive about their disability status are likely to have high self-esteem and vice versa. These individuals should fare well vocationally.

Social support was significantly correlated with all of the measures of employment success in the bivariate analyses. However, social support was not a significant predictor in the multivariate analyses. Social support also did not make a significant contribution to vocational success when other variables such as self-esteem and attitudes toward the disability were present. This finding was unexpected because of the strong impact of social support on adjustment to disability found in other studies (Belgrave & Walker, 1991a & b; Wilson, 1988). One possible explanation for why social support was not significant in the multivariate analyses (but was significant in the bivariate analyses) is that it is tied closely to self-esteem and attitudes toward the disability. Therefore, social support may not have made a contribution to explaining the variance after controlling for self-esteem and attitudes toward the disability. This finding suggests that social support may indirectly impact vocational success through its impact on self-esteem and attitudes toward disability.

The study supported Wallander's et al. (1989) model of risk and resistance factors in adaption of chronic illness and disability. The results of this study indicated that both risk and resistance factors accounted for successful employment outcomes. All of the resistance factors were significant in multivariate analyses. The risk factor was significant in two of the multivariate analyses. The current study provides support for the role of intrapersonal, socioecological, and stress-processing variables in this population of African Americans with disabilities.

SUMMARY

The purpose of this study was to identify factors and test a model of resistance and risk factors on employment outcomes of African Americans with disabilities. In doing so, we gained a better perspective of the target population.

Some of the findings on vocational variables are especially noteworthy. An overwhelming majority desired to work and a large percentage, 78%, felt they could work. These findings debunk the myth that persons who are unemployed do not want to work and are satisfied with receiving social services and unemployment benefits. This desire to work can be used to motivate the individual to acquire skills to enhance employability.

The results provide partial support for risk and resistance variables as predictors of employment outcomes. All three of the resistance factors and the one risk factor were related to employment outcomes in the bivariate analyses. Self-esteem (intrapersonal factor), beliefs about disability (stress-processing factor), perceived support (socioecological factor) and disability severity (risk factor) were related to both employment status and attitude toward employment.

Multivariate analyses allowed us to assess the unique contributions of each of the resistance and risk factors when all other factors were accounted for. The analysis performed with employment status as the outcome revealed that two of the resistance factors made unique and significant contributions (attitudes toward disability and self-esteem). Perceived capability to perform usual type of work was also significant. The analysis performed with attitude toward employment as the outcome variable yielded somewhat similar findings. Two of the resistance factors (beliefs about the disability and self-esteem) made unique contributions, along with the one risk factor (disability severity).

Although social support was significantly related to employment outcomes in the bivariate analyses, this factor did not emerge as a significant contributor when considered simultaneously with other variables. This finding suggests that social support may be more indirectly linked to employment through its influence on self-esteem, beliefs about disability, or other variables that were not tested in this study.

Vocational factors were significantly related to employment outcomes in bivariate analyses. Participants whose usual occupation was professional or blue-collar (in contrast with service or labor types of occupations) were more likely to be employed and to have more favorable attitudes toward work. Perceived capability to perform one's usual type of work and perceived ability to work were significantly associated with employment status. Respondents who felt they could perform the same type of work they had performed prior to becoming disabled were more likely to be employed and to have favorable work attitudes. Similarly respondents who felt they had the ability to work were more likely to be employed.

There are several implications that can be derived from the study findings. But first a cautionary note about the limitation of this study. Overall, study participants seemed to be faring better than the general population of African Americans with disabilities. A higher percentage were employed, with higher levels of education. All of the participants were recruited through a rehabilitation or medical facility or agency. Therefore, these individuals may be different from the population of persons who are not affiliated with a rehabilitation or medical facility. For example, they may have better access to rehabilitation services and may be more motivated to seek work.

Respondents were questioned by an interviewer who used a structured questionnaire. As such, responses were self-report and subject to the biases associated with any self-report data (i.e., socially desirability response set, unreliable recall, etc.).

With these limitations noted, we feel that the study helps us to understand and to subsequently develop better programs to increase positive employment outcomes for African Americans with disabilities. The finding that employment outcomes were better for those individuals who were capable of performing their usual type of work has an implication for the type of jobs that persons with disabilities seek. Efforts to redesign existing jobs or to assist persons in finding similar jobs may be more fruitful than training persons to do new and different jobs. It is likely that training and finding new jobs will be more costly than redesigning old jobs. Therefore, this finding has cost-saving implications.

The finding of the significant role of self-esteem and beliefs about the disability implies that programs that enhance self-esteem and positive beliefs about disability are important. Participatory programs that originate from the community with the active involvement of African Americans with disabilities in the planning, implementation, and evaluation are likely to be successful. Implicit in the development of such programs is that consumers support and empower each other. Research on social support is discussed in the next chapter. While this chapter focused on employment outcomes, the factors identified as important to employment are desirable for other adaptable behaviors such as good mental health and adaptive functioning in activities of daily living.

5

The Role of Social Support in Adaptive Functioning Among African Americans with Chronic Illnesses and Disabilities

As noted in previous chapters, several factors are expected to facilitate adaptive functioning among African Americans with disabilities. This chapter examines one socioenvironmental factor believed to facilitate outcomes for African Americans with disabilities. This factor is social support.

African Americans with disabilities are at increased risk of stress and subsequently negative functional outcomes (Manton, Patrick, & Johnson, 1987; McNeil, 1993). Social support may play an important role in reducing stress and facilitating adaptive functioning among these individuals. Social support has been found to be a significant factor in overall adjustment to disability, as well as adjustment in specific areas including employment (Belgrave & Walker, 1991a & b; Walker et al., 1995), mental

The study discussed in this chapter was supported by a grant (number MH46048) to Faye Z. Belgrave (Principal Investigator) from the National Institute of Mental Health. A revised version of this chapter was published earlier (Belgrave, F. Z., Davis, A., & Vajda, J. [1994]). An examination of social support source, type, and satisfaction among African Americans and White Americans with disabilities, *Journal of Social Behavior and Personality, 9*, 307–320). The authors would like to acknowledge the following individuals for their support in data collection: Drs. Robert Levin, Paul Kimmel, Beat von Albertini, and Joan Watson of George Washington University Hospital, DC, and Drs. Deborah Lewis and Sam Gordon at the National Rehabilitation Hospital, Washington, DC. Special thanks also to all persons who participated in the study.

health (Belgrave, 1991), and health decisions (Belgrave & Lewis, 1994) for African Americans with disabilities.

This chapter begins with a definition of social support and includes a discussion of conceptual and methodological issues that relate to understanding social support. This is followed by an overview of the literature on social support among African Americans, including how aspects of social support differ for African Americans and other ethnic groups. Research on the relationship between social support and selected outcomes for African Americans with disabilities is discussed next. A study that comprehensively examined several aspects of social support among African Americans with disabilities is then presented. The final part of the chapter discusses implications and recommendations for using social support for improving outcomes for African Americans.

WHAT IS SOCIAL SUPPORT?

According to Cobb (1976), social support is information from others that one is loved and cared for, esteemed and valued, and part of a network of communication and mutual obligations. Over the past three decades, there has been a voluminous amount of research showing that social support has both direct and buffering effects on outcomes across diverse domains (Cohen & McKay, 1984; Cohen, 1988; Cohen & Wills, 1985; Stroebe & Stroebe, 1997). These domains (among others) include mental and physical health, achievement and performance, and vocational and functional outcomes.

Direct Versus Buffering Effect of Social Support

The model of a direct effect of social support contends that social support has beneficial effects in all situations. That is, outcomes are expected to improve if social support is available. The buffering model regards social support as beneficial only for those experiencing stress. That is, social support will be beneficial only under stressful periods. This model assumes social support will not be beneficial for those without stressors. Cohen and Wills (1985) in their review of the research find evidence supporting both direct and buffering effects of social support. In a review of twenty-three studies, Kessler and McLeod (1985) found overwhelming support for the buffering hypothesis. Regardless of whether social support has a direct or a buffering effect, social support is believed to be especially beneficial for African Americans with disabilities, who may experience increased stress related to both disability and ethnic minority status in this country.

Conceptualization and Measurement of Social Support

In order to understand how social support is accessed and used among African Americans, it is helpful to understand how social support is conceptualized. Understanding the multidimensionality of the social support construct is useful when identifying the specific kinds of social support that may be most beneficial for African Americans.

Social support can be defined (and subsequently measured) along several dimensions. There are several topologies for conceptualizing support (Stroebe & Stroebe, 1997). *Support existence* is the presence or absence of a supportive relationship. *Network structure* concerns the providers of support. *Type or content of social support* refers to the function support provides. Questions pertaining to existence center around whether or not there is social support. Does social support exist? Is there an interpersonal relationship? Network structure is the set of relationships within which the recipient functions. Who are the providers of support? Social support may be personal or impersonal, provided by friends, relatives, and associates. Social support may be formal or informal. Type or content of social support refers to the type or the nature of social support and may include emotional, cognitive, and material support. Providing persons with information about a therapy regimen would be a form of cognitive support. Providing child-care assistance while the individual participated in a therapy session would be a form of material support. Giving comfort and reassurance as one is about to undergo a therapeutic procedure is a form of emotional support.

Other dimensions of support have been identified by others (Barrera, 1986; Gottlieb, 1983). One dimension is perceived versus enacted support. Here the distinction is made between whether or not the recipient of the support believes support to be provided versus whether or not someone actually does something to provide support (Barrera, 1986). A second dimension is social embeddedness. *Social embeddedness* refers to the connections that individuals have to significant others within their environments. As we have seen throughout this book, connections to others may be especially important to African Americans.

Another way of categorizing social support is whether or not it is functional or structural. Functional aspects of social support are concerned with the function or the role served by social support (i.e., what is actually gained or believed to be gained). Structural aspects of support are concerned with the integration of the person within a support network. Perceived and enacted aspects of social support would be reflected in the functional aspects of social support. Social embeddedness would reflect the structural aspects of social support.

In understanding the contribution of social support, it is necessary to recognize the multidimensionality of support in that a particular aspect of support will be most beneficial if matched to the needs of the individual. For example, for a person with very limited financial resources, material support in the form of transportation and child-care assistance may be most beneficial. However, for a person adapting to a recently acquired disability, emotional and cognitive support may be especially helpful. Another consideration for African Americans is the cultural congruence of the support received and given. Social support may not be beneficial if it is provided in an impersonal and disjointed manner. The authenticity of the provider of support may be a factor in whether or not support is accepted by African Americans.

Although social support in general is beneficial, the social support may not have beneficial effects in all situations (Cohen, 1988; Cohen & McKay, 1984; Schumaker & Brownell, 1984). As noted, in order for social support to be most beneficial, the source and type of support must be matched to the needs of the person and the situation. If the individual with a disability has wealth, material support may not be necessary. Informational and cognitive support may be more important. If on the other hand, the individual is hungry and has no food, all the love, warmth, and information in the world will not help.

A key theme throughout this book is that there are cultural values and beliefs among African Americans that may influence aspects of social support that is accessed, provided, and used.

Model of Social Support, Stress, and Outcomes for African Americans with Disabilities

A proposed model for understanding the role of social support in outcomes for African Americans with disabilities is shown in Figure 5.1. The model depicted has been adapted from various models of stress and social support (see Anderson, 1991; Cohen, 1988; Cohen & McKay, 1984).

As seen in Figure 5.1, both internal and external conditions can contribute to stress. For the person with a disability, these may include the functional limitations imposed by the disabling conditions, poor socioenvironmental conditions (Anderson, 1991; Myers, 1983) as well as racist and oppressive attitudes held by some in rehabilitation and medical settings. These stressors may negatively impact physiological processes through impaired immune functioning. Additionally, these stressors may interfere with the person's ability to make healthy decisions and to engage in healthy behaviors. Attention to diet or a rehabilitation regimen may be forgone during stressful periods. The impact of stress then may lead to poor outcomes across several domains—poor vocational and functional outcomes and impaired mental and physical health.

Social support may buffer the perceived stress at two points in the causal link between stress and outcomes. First, support may mediate

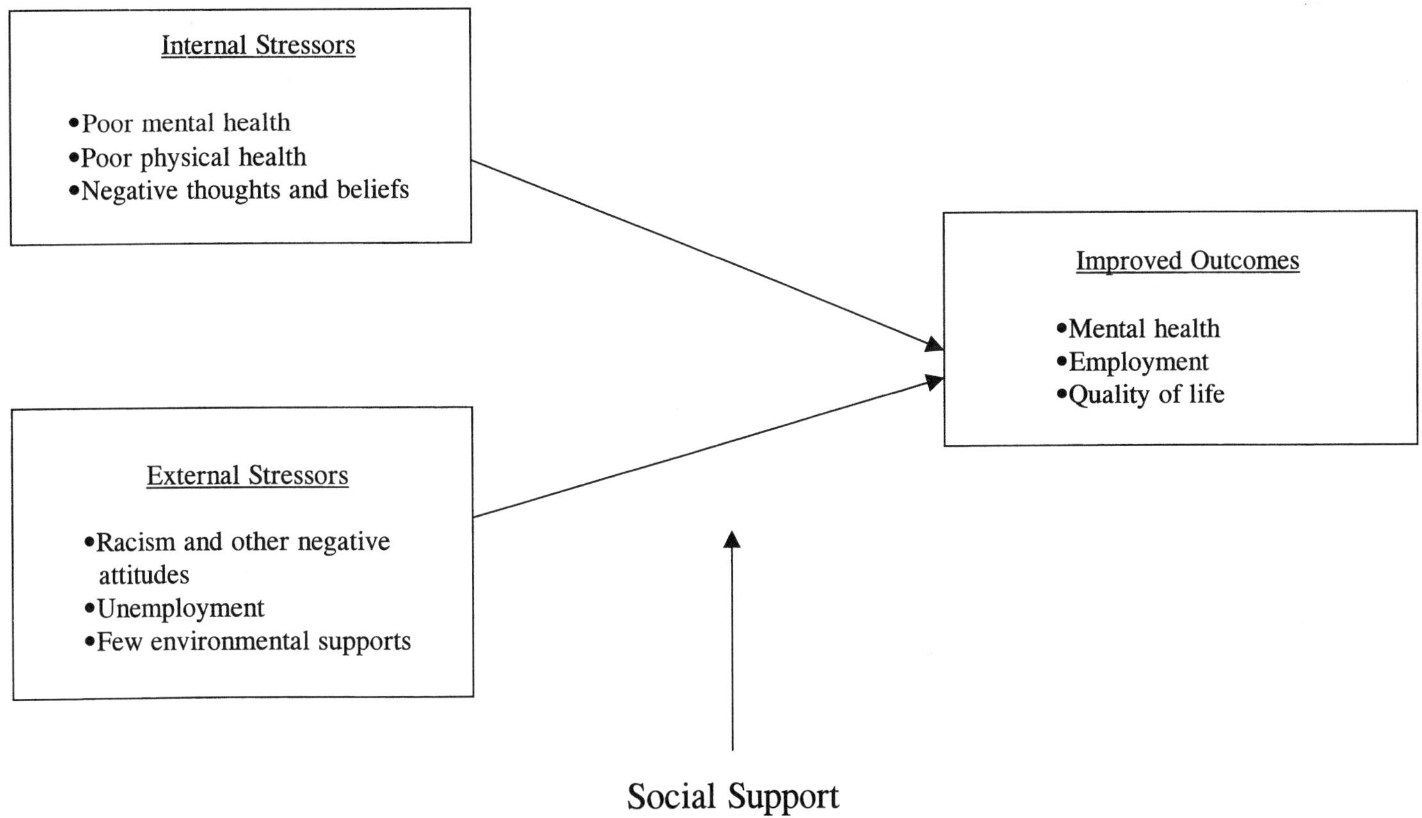

Figure 5.1
Model of Social Support, Stress, and Outcomes Among African Americans with Disabilities

between the stressor and the reaction to the stress by minimizing or preventing a negative stress appraisal response (i.e., impaired physiological reaction or poor health decisions). The perception that support is available may alter the perception of the stressor or augment the person's belief that the stressor can be coped with. Second, support may intervene between the reaction or the experience of stress and the negative outcome by changing maladaptive responses. For example, support in the form of the rent being paid or assistance in finding a job may facilitate vocational outcomes. Receiving emotional support in the form of love, reassurance, and concern may improve mental health. For African Americans, cognitive and emotional support from similar others may buffer the impact of an oppressive environment.

Cultural values and beliefs are believed to exert an influence on how stressors are perceived and how support is accessed and used. For example, spiritual beliefs may mediate the perception of an event or condition as being stressful if it is seen within a spiritual framework. Faith can contribute positively to acceptance of one's life circumstance. A communal orientation may influence the type of support that is provided, accessed, and used. Support may be expected, valued, and used from others within the extended family and community.

SOCIAL SUPPORT AMONG AFRICAN AMERICANS

There have been a number of studies which have investigated social support among African Americans. These studies have examined social support among elderly African Americans (Mindel & Wright, 1982; Smith-Ruiz, 1985; Taylor & Chatters, 1986), African American adolescents (Cauce, Felner, & Primavera, 1982; Coates, 1985) low-income African Americans (Ball, 1983) and African Americans at risk for health problems (Dressler, Dos-Santos, & Vileri, 1986; Stephens, 1985).

Dressler, Dos-Santos, and Primavera (1986) examined the impact of social support on stress and depression using a sample of 122 African American households from a rural southern setting. They were interested in determining whether or not support network could act as a buffer against stress related to depression. The results of the study showed a buffering effect of social support on stress for males, but not for females. Brown and Gary (1987) studied the impact of stress and social support on health using an urban African American sample. They were interested in determining whether the social support relationship varied for psychological and physical health. Psychological health was measured using a depression scale, and physical health was assessed with a single question asking subjects to rate their health as excellent, good, fair, or poor. Stress was measured using Holmes and Rahe's inventory of stressful life events. Social support was assessed by looking at the structure of the social network, (i.e., number of relatives living close by, number of confidants, and number of close friends). Brown and Gary found that social support had a buffering effect on the mental health of females, but not of males. African American females with high perceived social support experienced fewer symptoms and had a less dramatic rise in mental distress as the number of stressful life events increased.

In a doctoral dissertation, Chase (1992) surveyed 205 African American college students. She found that perceived availability of support from both family, kin, and others buffered the impact of stress on adjustment for these students. That is, those students who were experiencing high stress were able to adapt better to college when social support was available than when it was not available. In summary, the literature suggests that social support favorably impacts outcomes across several populations and domains for African Americans.

Differences in Social Support Among African Americans and Other Ethnic Groups

Several studies have focused on the nature of social support and dimensions of social support that differ for African Americans and other ethnic groups. Studies have shown that compared to White Americans, African Americans are more likely to use more natural support systems and informal types of social support from family, friends, and the church (Endo, 1984; Mindel, 1980; Mindel & Wright, 1982; Neighbors & Jackson, 1984; Raymond, Rhoads, & Raymond, 1980; Taylor & Chatters, 1986). In one study Raymond, Rhoads, & Raymond (1980) found that African Americans placed more importance on family in sharing experiences and in giving and receiving help than did Whites. Mindel (1980) found African Americans to have more households of kin in the community and to be in more contact with extended family members than did White Americans. Furthermore, the results of the study by Mindel show that African Americans use support differently than Mexican Americans and Anglo Americans. African Americans use their kin in a more instrumental fashion as a mutual aid-and-support system than these other ethnic groups. Cauce et al. (1982), in a study of Black adolescents, found that they rely more heavily on family support than either Hispanic or White adolescents.

In fact, the use of informal systems of support has been central to the survival and adaptation of African Americans in the United States. Given limited resources and often oppressive environments, African Americans have had to rely upon one another for support. Thomas, Milburn, Brown, and Gary (1988) write, "the utility of these (informal) support systems to mitigate against the deleterious effects of psychological trauma is of critical importance to the Black community since it is apparent that a sizeable proportion of its population lives under stressful conditions. Furthermore, since research suggests that Black adults are often reluctant to seek assistance from mental health facilities, informal support systems may play a key role in the coping process" (p. 36).

Support Specificity. As noted earlier, the beneficial aspects of social support may be enhanced by matching the appropriate type of support to the needs of the person. The literature suggests the amount (i.e., number of persons who provide support) of social support may differentially relate to outcomes for different ethnic groups. Griffith (1985) found the amount of social support was related to psychological distress for non-Whites but not for Whites. Correspondingly, the type of support may differentially relate to outcomes for different ethnic minority groups. Strogatz and James (1986) found low instrumental support was associated with increased hypertension for African Americans, but not for White Americans. Emotional support was not correlated with hypertension for either group. In a study of ethnic minority rehabilitation clients (of which the majority were African American), Walker et al. (1995) found that employment efficacy was positively correlated with support from the family, but not from professionals. This study suggests that among African Americans support from the family and kin may be more beneficial than support from other sources. The literature suggests that in order for social support to be effective, the amount, type, and provider must be matched to the needs of the person. Cultural congruence is one factor to consider in this matching.

THE ROLE OF SOCIAL SUPPORT IN OUTCOMES OF AFRICAN AMERICANS WITH DISABILITIES

Several studies have investigated the role of social support on outcomes of African Americans with disabilities. Some of these studies have been conducted by the author and are reviewed below.

Belgrave, Lewis, & Scott (1994) investigated the role of social support on health care adherence in a population of African Americans with sickle cell disease and diabetes. One hundred twenty-seven persons (49 with sickle cell disease and 78 with diabetes) completed a questionnaire that assessed the availability of emotional, cognitive, and material support. Health care adherence regarding appointments and health behaviors (i.e., diet, exercise, regular blood pressure tests, taking medication) were also obtained through this self-report questionnaire. The results of this study indicated a significant correlation between the availability of social support and health care adherence. Social support was related to whether or not the person kept his or her medical appointments and whether or not the person engaged in good health behaviors such as eating nutritiously, having regular checkups, and having blood pressure monitored.

The findings of this study are consistent with that of studies using non–African American populations that have shown a positive benefit of social support on compliance. Social support may assist persons in carrying out health care recommendations they could not do alone. For example, eating behaviors may be determined by the food that is bought and prepared within the house. Adherence to medical appointments may be contingent upon the availability of transportation. Finally the encouragement and concern of significant others may encourage the person to take care of themself. The support of others within the family may be especially needed by African Americans, whose family unit may be very interdependent.

In another study the author was interested in the influence of social support on employment status, that is, whether or not the person was employed (Belgrave & Walker, 1991b). In this study social support was included as a variable, along with other psychological and demographic variables. The availability of emotional, cognitive, and material support was assessed, along with employment status, via a questionnaire.

The results of this study indicated that a significant percentage of the variance in employment status could be explained by the variables in the study. Social support was a significant contributor—in fact, social support and source of transportation were the only two variables that made significant contributions to explaining employment. Persons who reported high availability of social support and those who had cars (or private vehicles) were more likely to be employed than those without social support and without access to private vehicles. The finding of this study highlights the contribution of social support as a contributor to an important outcome—employment.

In a related study, Walker, Belgrave, Jarama, Ukawuilulu, and Rackley (1995) investigated the relationship between the availability of social support and employment efficacy among ethnic minority individuals with disabilities. The majority (68%) of these individuals were African Americans. The relationship between social support and job efficacy was examined, and job efficacy was defined as beliefs that employment could be secured and maintained.

Participants included forty-four clients of rehabilitation agencies. They were administered questionnaires that obtained measures of social support and job efficacy at two points in time. The results showed a significant correlation between social support and job efficacy at both time periods. That is, respondents who reported that social support was available at time one and six weeks later (time two) were more likely to have favorable beliefs in their ability to obtain and keep a job. Of particular relevance here was the finding that the availability of support from professional sources was negatively correlated with job efficacy. That is, respondents who reported receiving more support from professional sources were less likely to believe that they could obtain and maintain employment. On the other hand, the availability of support from family, that is, parents, was positively correlated with job efficacy. One interpretation of these findings is that those who need more support from professionals are less functional. However, an alternative interpretation, consistent with the thesis of this chapter, is that social support from the family is more culturally congruent for this population.

Another study by Belgrave (1991) was conducted to explore the influence of social support in an interpersonal domain—acceptance of disability. The study was concerned with the extent to which social support along with other variables (i.e., self-esteem, locus of control, disability severity, and demographic variables) contributed to acceptance of the disability. Data were gathered from 170 African Americans with disabilities. Disabilities included (a) speech and hearing impairments, (b) orthopedic impairments, (c) mental illness and substance abuse, and (d) other impairments.

The results of a regression analysis indicated that three of the psychosocial variables—perception of disability severity, social support, and self-esteem—were significant contributors and accounted for 50% of the variance in explaining acceptance of disability in the study's sample. None of the demographic variables were significantly related to acceptance of disability. The results of this study suggest that social support may be more influential than socioeconomical factors such as education and income as a contributor to employment.

The finding of the contribution of social support to acceptance of disability is underscored because acceptance of disability is an important outcome. When a person accepts and feels comfortable with having a disability, self-esteem and overall mental health will be positive.

In summary, the research has shown a positive benefit of social support across diverse outcomes for African Americans with disabilities. Adherence to health care and rehabilitation recommendations can be expected to be facilitated by the availability of social support. Adherence to appropriate rehabilitation regimens should facilitate mental and physical health outcomes. Given the lower participation of African Americans in rehabilitation programs, increased social support may be especially beneficial in this regard. Social support also has been associated with improved employment and mental health outcomes. These outcomes impact the quality of life, and efforts to improve these outcomes can be targeted in interventions.

While research has shown social support to be generally beneficial for African Americans with disabilities, we know less about the mechanism by which this support works. An understanding of the mechanism is necessary to develop programs and services that use social support to improve outcomes. For example, who are the providers of social support for African Americans with disabilities? Are some types of support more beneficial than others? Does support relate to functional outcomes, and does the relationship between social support and functional outcomes differ for African Americans and other ethnic groups with disabilities?

These and other questions were addressed in a study conducted by the author and colleagues (Belgrave, Davis, & Vadja, 1994) on aspects of social support among African Americans. Funding for this study was provided by the National Institute of Mental Health. The study was developed to comprehensively examine the nature of social support among African Americans with disabilities.

AN EXAMINATION OF SOCIAL SUPPORT AMOUNT, SOURCE AND TYPE AMONG AFRICAN AMERICANS WITH DISABILITIES

The primary purpose of this study was to determine how social support differed for African Americans and other ethnic minority groups with disabilities (Belgrave, Davis, & Vadja, 1994). The study examined differences between African Americans and White Americans with disabilities regarding social support amount, source (i.e., provider), type, and satisfaction. An additional purpose was to determine whether or not social support differentially related to two outcomes (i.e., mental health status and adaptive functioning) for African Americans and White Americans. Mental health status and adaptive functioning were chosen as outcome (dependent) variables because of their impact on the quality of life for persons with disabilities. The following questions were addressed:

1. Are there differences between African Americans and Whites in the amount of support overall and from different sources (i.e, do African Americans and White Americans report differences in the total number of persons who provide support as well as the number of family, kin, friends, and others who provide support)?
2. Are there ethnic differences in level of satisfaction with support overall as well as satisfaction with support from family, kin, friends, and others?
3. Are there ethnic differences in satisfaction with support overall and satisfaction with emotional, cognitive, and instrumental types of support?
4. Are there gender differences regarding who provides support for African Americans and White Americans?

5. Does satisfaction with support relate to mental health and adaptive functioning, and is this relationship different for African Americans and White Americans?

Methods and Procedures

Participants. Participants were 80 African Americans and Whites with disabilities. In this study, a disability was defined as an impairment that causes a restriction in activities of daily living at home, work, or within the community. Forty-eight (58.7%) were African American and thirty-two (42.5%) were Whites. Forty-six were males and thirty-six were females. Ages ranged from 21 to 85, with a mean age of 52. Regarding marital status, 46.8% were married and 53.2% were not married. Participants' education ranged from some elementary school to graduate school.

Participants were recruited from three sites: (1) a rehabilitation hospital, (2) a rehabilitation unit at an acute care hospital, and (3) a renal outpatient clinic affiliated with the same acute care hospital. Twenty-five percent reported their primary disabling condition as stroke; 31.3% reported spinal cord injury; 22.5% reported renal disease; and 21.2% reported some other disability. Of the participants, 72.5% had one or more hospitalizations over the previous year, and 27.5% had not been hospitalized over the previous year.

Overall, the level of disability among the participants could be described as moderate to severe. Only 35% of the participants were employed. On the question, "overall, how severely disabled do you think you are?" 63.5% of the participants indicated that they were moderately to very severely disabled. The scale ranged from slightly disabled to very severely disabled.

Measures. The Arizona Social Support Interview Schedule (ASSIS) (Barrera, 1981; Barrera, Sandler, & Ramsay, 1981) was used to measure social support source, number of persons who provide support, satisfaction with support, and type of support. The respondent is asked to provide the names or initials of persons who provide support across six situations (e.g., "If you wanted to talk to someone about things that are very personal and private, who are the people you would talk to?" The respondent is then asked to indicate whether or not the amount of support was adequate on a scale that ranges from 1 (a lot more support needed) to 5 (support was just about right). The six situations capture emotional, cognitive, and instrumental support. The respondent is also asked to indicate whether or not the persons listed are family, kin, friend, or other and whether they are male or female.

Test-retest reliability of the ASSIS was assessed on a sample of college students and was adequate (Barrera, 1981). The internal consistency of the ASSIS using a sample of African American college students was .84 (Chase, 1992).

Several social support scores were derived for this study: (a) total number of persons providing support across the six situations (computed by totaling the number of persons listed for each situation); (b) total number of persons who provide support who are family, kin, friend, and other (computed by summing the number of persons listed for each source of support); (c) overall satisfaction with support (computed by first obtaining an average score for each question on the level of support and then averaging these scores across the six questions); (d) total amount of each type of social support (i.e., emotional, cognitive and instrumental; computed by totaling the number of persons listed for each type of support); and (e) satisfaction with type (i.e., emotional, instrumental, and cognitive) of support (computed by averaging the values (1–5) on whether or not the amount of support was about right for type of support).

The Beck Depression Inventory was used to assess depression which was used as an indicator of mental health status (Beck, Steer, & Garbin, 1988). The 22-item Beck is a commonly used scale for measuring level of depression in medical and nonmedical populations and has demonstrated reliability as well as concurrent validity with other measures of depression and construct validity with psychological, behavioral, and attitudinal variables related to depression. Cronbach's reliability coefficient for the study sample was .81.

The adaptive behavior subscale of the Personal Capacities Questionnaire (PCQ) was used to measure adaptive functioning. This subscale consists of six items in which the respondent indicates on a scale from 0 (most adaptive) to 3 (least adaptive) his or her level of adaptive behaviors. The adaptive behavior items assess the client's perceptions of his or her work habits, awareness of abilities and limitations, getting along with supervisors and coworkers, judgment, desire to work, and initiative and problem-solving ability. The PCQ is the client self-report version of the Functional Assessment Inventory (FAI) (Crew & Alhelstan, 1984), which is completed by a rehabilitation specialist. An item by item translation of the FAI was used to develop the PCQ. The FAI has adequate validity and reliability (Crew & Alhelstan, 1984).

Procedure. Participants were recruited in two ways. In the first, letters were sent to persons who had been discharged from the rehabilitation hospital over the previous twelve months. They were asked to contact project staff if interested in participating in the study. Second, some participants were met by an interviewer while they were receiving treatment at the hospital or clinic and were asked if they were interested in participating in the study. An appointment for data collection was scheduled for a future time. An African American interviewer collected data from African American participants and a White interviewer collected data from White participants. Both interviewers were female.

Prior to the data collection session, participants were contacted by phone by the interviewers, and participation was confirmed. Participants were administered questionnaires at a mutually agreed-upon time and place by the participant and the interviewer. Data collection sessions were generally scheduled for participants before or after medical follow-up appointments at the hospital facilities.

After signing a consent form, each participant was given a questionnaire packet and asked to complete it. The interviewer was nearby and available if there were questions or if reading assistance was required. It took participants approximately 1.5 hours to complete the questionnaire. Participants were thanked and provided a payment incentive upon completion of the questionnaires.

Results

Descriptive Statistics on Social Support Variables. Descriptive statistics on social support variables for African American and White participants are shown in Tables 5.1 and 5.2. Across the six questions, African Americans reported 21.3 persons who provide support, and White Americans reported 24.3 persons who provide support. The source of support most frequently reported for both groups was family, followed by friends. Both groups listed relatively few in the "other" support category. The satisfaction level with support was moderately high for both groups; scores of 4.5 and 4.3 (out of a high score of 5.0) were reported for the African Americans and Whites respectively.

Tests of Research Questions. A variety of statistical analyses were computed in order to address the research questions. In order to address research question one, a multiple analysis of variance (MANOVA) was computed to examine differences in the number of persons who provide support overall and for family, kin, friends, and others for African Americans and White Americans. These were the dependent variables. Ethnicity was the independent variable. The MANOVA was marginally significant ($p = .06$). Univariate analyses revealed that only number of kin was significantly different for African Americans than whites ($p < .01$). African Americans reported significantly more kin than did Whites (2.71 versus .84). None of the other measures of amounts of sources of support were significantly different for African Americans and Whites.

The second research question regarding differences in satisfaction with overall support and sources of support was addressed by computing a series of independent sample *t*-tests. Scores for overall satisfaction and satisfaction from family, kin, friends, and others were dependent variables; ethnicity was the independent variable. A significant finding was

Table 5.1
Descriptive Statistics (Mean, Standard Deviation, and Range) on Social Support Variables for African Americans and Whites

Number of Persons	African Americans	Whites
Total who provide support	21.3	24.3
	11.0	15.6
	(6-50)	(4-71)
Family who provide support	11.8	12.4
	8.5	11.0
	(0-35)	(0-42)
Kin who provide support	2.7	.8
	3.1	3.3
	(0-11)	(0-18)
Friends who provide support	6.3	9.8
	8.4	11.2
	(0-35)	(0-53)
Others who provide support	1.2	1.3
	2.4	2.8
	(0-12)	(0-14)
Emotional support	6.9	8.0
	4.4	5.1
	(0-20)	(2-20)
Instrumental support	7.2	8.3
	4.5	5.7
	(1-23)	(0-23)
Cognitive support	2.5	1.4
	1.9	1.5
	(0-8)	(0-7)
Males who provide support	8.17	12.06
	5.19	8.22
	(0-22)	(0-36)
Females who provide support	13.32	12.25
	10.02	11.26
	(2-46)	(0-48)

Table 5.2
Descriptive Statistics (Mean, Standard Deviation, and Range) on Support Satisfaction Variables for African Americans and Whites with Disabilities

	African Americans	Whites
Average satisfaction with support	4.5 .62 (2-5)	4.3 .95 (1-5)
Satisfaction with support from family	4.5 .73 (2-5)	4.3 .91 (1-5)
Satisfaction with support from kin	4.8 .23 (3-5)	3.8 1.2 (2-5)
Satisfaction with support from friend	4.5 .87 (1-5)	4.2 1.3 (1-5)
Satisfaction with support from other	4.3 1.1 (1-5)	3.7 .60 (1-5)
Satisfaction with emotional support	4.5 .98 (1-5)	4.2 1.0 (1-5)
Satisfaction with instrumental support	4.7 .64 (1-5)	4.5 .92 (1-5)
Satisfaction with cognitive support	4.7 .60 (1-5)	4.3 1.1 (1-5)
Satisfaction with support from males	4.5 .75 (1-5)	4.2 1.1 (1-5)
Satisfaction with support from females	4.5 .75 (2-5)	4.6 .87 (1-5)

revealed for kin only. African Americans reported higher levels of satisfaction with support received from kin (4.8 versus 3.8) than whites ($p < .001$).

The third question was concerned with whether or not there were differences in the level of satisfaction overall and for emotional, instrumental, and cognitive types of support. A MANOVA was computed, with scores for overall satisfaction and satisfaction with emotional, instrumental, and cognitive support as the dependent variables and ethnicity as the dependent variable. The result of the MANOVA approached significance ($p = .10$). The univariate test revealed a significant difference regarding satisfaction with cognitive support ($p < .03$). African Americans were more satisfied with cognitive support than Whites (mean = 4.7 versus 4.3). A marginally significant difference was found for emotional support ($p < = .08$), with African Americans also reporting higher levels of satisfaction with emotional support than Whites.

The fourth research question was concerned with gender differences regarding providers of support. A series of *t*-tests was computed with ethnicity as the independent variable and amount of support and satisfaction with support received from both females and males as the dependent variables. White Americans reported that significantly more males provided support than African Americans ($p < .02$). Whites reported an average of 12 males, compared to African Americans, who reported an average of 8 males. There were no differences regarding satisfaction with support from males or females.

The fifth question was concerned with whether or not social support was related to two outcome measures (i.e., depression and adaptive functioning) and whether or not social support was differentially related to outcomes for the two groups. Four MANOVAs were computed to address this question, with measures of depression and adaptive functioning as dependent variables and ethnicity and social support as independent variables. Interactions between ethnicity and social support were computed to test for whether or not social support differentially related to outcomes for African Americans and Whites. Only analyses with significant results are reported. A MANOVA tested for the effects of (a) ethnicity, (b) satisfaction with support (overall), and (c) the interaction between ethnicity and satisfaction with support on depression. The results of this analysis revealed a significant effect for support satisfaction ($p < .009$). High social support satisfaction was associated with lower levels of depression ($r = -.28$).

An additional analysis tested for effects of variables on adaptive functioning. This analysis tested for the effects of (a) ethnicity, (b) number of persons who provide support, and (c) the interaction between ethnicity and number of persons who provide support on adaptive functioning. The results of this analysis showed a marginally significant effect for ethnicity ($p < .06$). Adaptive functioning among African Americans was not as favorable as that among Whites (mean = 2.3 versus .83—with lower scores denoting better functioning). There were no significant effects for amount of support nor interaction.

SUMMARY AND DISCUSSION

The primary purpose of this study was to examine aspects of social support among African Americans with disabilities and to determine if they differ from Whites. Another purpose was to determine how social support relates to outcomes for the two ethnic groups. A cautionary note regarding the generality of the study findings is necessary. The sample was relatively small (only 80 participants) and was recruited from medical settings. The relatively small sample size did not allow for an assessment of other factors that may have accounted for differences between the two groups, (i.e., type of disability, socioeconomic status, recruitment setting, etc.). Additional research using larger samples more representative of all persons with disabling conditions is needed.

The findings support literature that suggests that African Americans are more likely than Whites to use certain kinds of support systems, such as from the family and kin (Endo, 1984; Mindel & Wright, 1982; Neighbors & Jackson, 1984; Raymond, Rhoads, & Raymond, 1980; Taylor & Chatters, 1986). Although there were no differences between the two groups in the number of family members or friends who provide support, there were differences regarding the number of kin who provide support. Among this sample of African Americans, the distinction between family and kin may not have been as great as for Whites. The finding that African Americans (compared to Whites) relied upon a larger number of kin to provide support is also consistent with the literature on extended African American families. The extended African American family has been identified as important in the maintenance of mental and physical health (McAdoo, 1993). The extended family may serve as a buffer against stress for African Americans with disabilities. Not only were African Americans more likely to identify a larger number of kin who provided support; they were also more satisfied with support from kin than White Americans. Perhaps support relationships from kin are expected and valued among African Americans to a greater extent than among White Americans.

African Americans are less likely to utilize rehabilitation services than White Americans and are less likely to express satisfaction with these services (Belgrave & Walker, 1991a). Family and kin providers of support may fulfill support functions usually fulfilled by rehabilitation professionals.

The findings also indicated that African Americans were significantly more likely than Whites to report feeling satisfied with cognitive support. African Americans were also more likely than Whites to report satisfaction with emotional support and this difference approached significance. No differences were found regarding material support. Perhaps cognitive support (providing advice and information) and emotional support (providing reassurance, concern, and love) are easier types of support for African Americans to provide, given their relative lack of material resources. That is, African Americans may not have money or materialistic things to give, but they do find the time to provide information, show concern, and give reassurance. Concurrently cognitive and emotional forms of support may be the types of support that are valued by African Americans with disabilities, who may need reassurance and advice from significant others more than Whites. As noted, African Americans with disabilities may be less likely to have access to and use support from professionals (Belgrave & Walker, 1991b).

One purpose of this study was to determine whether or not the amount and satisfaction with social support was differentially related to mental health and adaptive behaviors for African Americans and White Americans. The analyses revealed that ethnicity did not mediate the relationship between social support and mental health and adaptive behaviors. That is, the nature of the relationship between social support and mental health and adaptive functioning did not differ for African Americans and Whites. However, the analyses did reveal a main effect for social support satisfaction on a mental health outcome (i.e., depression). High levels of satisfaction with social support were associated with lower levels of depression. This finding is consistent with previous literature that has shown a positive benefit of social support satisfaction for African Americans and other ethnic groups with disabilities (Belgrave, 1991; Belgrave, Walker, & Asbury, 1995).

While satisfaction with support was significantly related to mental health outcomes, the amount of support was not. These findings suggest social support satisfaction might be more influential than amount of support or size of one's support network for improving outcomes. That is, the amount of support or the number of persons in a person's support network may be less important than being satisfied with the support that is provided.

A marginally significant effect for ethnicity on adaptive functioning was also found. African Americans were more likely to report less favorable adaptive functioning than White Americans. This finding is consistent with previous literature that reports that functional impairment is greater for African Americans than Whites (McNeil, 1993).

The findings from this study are important because they extend the literature on social support providers to a population that has not been studied previously—African Americans with disabilities. Although this population may experience increased stress because of ethnic minority and disability status, there has been limited research on African Americans with disabilities. The finding of differences regarding providers of support has both theoretical and practical value. Theoretically the study contributes to the literature on social support because it underscores the importance of ethnicity and culture as a factor in understanding who provides support, specifically to a population of persons with disabilities. Additional support resources from those outside of the immediate family, that is, kin, may be an especially useful resource among African Americans. Given the historical economic disadvantaged status of African Americans, support resources from extended family and kin may be especially needed. From an applied perspective, the findings suggest an understanding of African Americans with disabilities would be facilitated by understanding who provides support to these individuals.

IMPLICATIONS AND RECOMMENDATIONS

The development of programs to teach persons how to access social support is one practical consideration from the research reviewed in this chapter. One specific application would be to teach persons how to access satisfactory social support relationships. This would seem to be true for both African Americans and Whites with disabilities. Given the differences regarding providers of support, one might wish to consider this when planning programs and services. African Americans and Whites could learn to access different sources of support with kin perhaps included for African Americans, but not for Whites. One implication here is that persons can be trained to identify and access supportive resources within family, kin, and community networks. Guidelines for implementing a social support intervention are provided in chapter 7.

6

Intrapersonal Resources for Increasing Adaptive Functioning Among African Americans with Disabilities and Chronic Illnesses

As discussed in the previous two chapters, social support has beneficial aspects for improving outcomes among African Americans with disabilities and chronic illnesses. Social support is an external resource that can be used to improve adaptive coping and adjustment. Intrapersonal, or inner, resources is the focus of this chapter. In it intrapersonal resources are conceptualized as psychological resources, that is, those factors which reside within the individual. These intrapersonal, or psychological, resources are believed to be just as important as external resources in one's ability to cope with and adapt to a disability or chronic illness. An understanding of these resources and how they can be used to facilitate adaptive functioning is the focus of this chapter.

Several intrapersonal resources or psychological factors could be discussed in this chapter. These include underlying personality dispositions such as self-esteem, optimism, hardiness, achievement motivation, and resiliency. Two intrapersonal factors that seem relevant for understanding and providing an appropriate framework for improving outcomes among African Americans with chronic illness and disability were selected for discussion. These are (a) self-efficacy and psychological control and (b) coping patterns. Both intrapersonal factors are based on cognitions. *Cognitions* are our thoughts, feelings, beliefs, and ways of viewing the world, others, and ourselves. Cognitions have a pervasive influence on how we experience the world. Both self-efficacy and coping patterns are related to social support insofar as their presence or absence seems to be linked to the presence or absence of social support. (This point will be expanded upon later in this chapter.)

Understanding the role of these two intrapersonal resources on adaptive functioning of African Americans with chronic illnesses and disabilities is an important first step in developing programs to improve functioning. Of note is that these intrapersonal resources are within the control of the individual, and individuals can learn to access and use them. This approach is empowering insofar as the impetus for change comes from within the individual.

The discussion that follows provides an overview of research and literature on (a) self-efficacy theory and other theories of psychological control and (b) coping. These two theories will be discussed with considerations toward their applications for improving outcomes for African Americans with chronic illnesses and disabilities. Recommendations for improving self-efficacy and for increasing adaptive coping patterns will be provided in chapter 8.

SELF-EFFICACY THEORY AND PSYCHOLOGICAL CONTROL

Self-efficacy theory provides a useful framework for understanding and improving behaviors across diverse populations, including African Americans with disabilities. Self-efficacy theory is derived from social learning theory and is concerned with whether or not a person believes he/she can accomplish a desired outcome (Bandura, 1977, 1986). According to Bandura, self-efficacious beliefs are central to achieving desired behaviors. Beliefs about one's capabilities affect what a person chooses to do, how much effort is put into a task, and how long a person will persevere in the face of difficulties. Self-efficacious beliefs also impact the person's emotional reactions to situations. Under conditions of high self-efficacy, a person's mental health is likely to remain positive, even under stressful and aversive conditions. Under conditions of low self-efficacy, mental health may deteriorate, even when environmental conditions are favorable. Self-efficacy has been shown to contribute to favorable outcomes across several domains including achievement (Garland, Weinberg, Bruya, & Jackson, 1988; Hackett & Betz, 1996; Taylor, Locke, Lee, & Gist, 1984); health promotion and illness prevention (Bandura, 1990; Covington & Omelich, 1992; Ewart, 1996; Kalisky, Rubison, Laurence, & Levy, 1990; Stretcher, De Vellis, Becker, & Rosenstock, 1986; Weitzel & Waller, 1990); pain management (Dolce, 1987; Hoffman & Loring, 1992; O'Leary, Shoor, Lorig, & Holman, 1988); and mental health (DiClemente, Fairhurst, & Piotrowsky, 1996).

There have been several investigations of self-efficacy among medical populations and among persons with disabilities (Allegrante, MacKenzie, & Robbins, 1991; Cicerone, 1991; Ewart, 1992, 1996; Gattuso, Litt, & Fitzgerald, 1992; Maddux, 1996; Mitchell, Brodwin, & Benoit, 1990; O'Leary, Shoor, Lorig, & Holman, 1988; Patridge & Johnson, 1989; Taal, Rasker, Seydel, & Weigman, 1993; Terry, 1992; Wassen, 1992). Generally, these studies have found a beneficial impact of self-efficacy on outcomes, with self-efficacious beliefs associated with better functional outcomes (O'Leary et al., 1988; Schiaffino, Revenson, & Gibofsky, 1991; Taal et al., 1993), decreased pain (Dolce, 1987; Jensen, Turner, & Romano, 1991; Taal et al., 1993) and increased social and psychological competence (Cicerone, 1991; Schiaffino & Revenson, 1992).

Research by Taal, Rasker, Seydel, and Weigman (1993) on self-management of disability and pain and adherence to health recommendations among persons with arthritis found that difficulties in these areas were related to low self-efficacy expectations about coping with arthritis. The authors suggested that patient education should strengthen self-efficacy beliefs along with using support as a motivational factor.

O'Leary, Shoor, Lorig, and Holman (1988) used a cognitive-behavioral intervention to increase self-efficacy among persons with rheumatoid arthritis. In this study, participants were assigned to either a control group or an intervention group. In the control group, participants received a self-help booklet; in the intervention group, participants were taught skills in managing stress, pain, and disease symptoms. Participants in the intervention group experienced reduced pain and improved psychological functioning. Moreover, the degree to which people improved was correlated with the degree of self-efficacy enhancement, suggesting increases in perceived self-efficacy were responsible for the effectiveness of the intervention.

In a review of the literature on self-efficacy and myocardial infraction (MCI), Ewart (1996) argues that self-efficacy theory provides a useful framework for understanding recovery from MCI. According to this author, self-efficacious beliefs influence behavioral responses to MCI (e.g., more exercise, stress management, improved diet). These in turn lead to better physical recovery.

Thompson, Gil, Abrams, and Phillips (1992) found that positive psychosocial adjustment was associated with lower levels of perceived daily stress, and higher efficacy expectations regarding illness tasks. Individuals who had high efficacy beliefs that they could handle illness-related tasks had more positive psychosocial adjustment. These authors also found that psychosocial factors accounted for a more significant percentage of the variance in psychological adjustment than demographic or illness parameter variables such as sex, age, socioeconomic status, or illness severity.

There has also been some research on self-efficacy among African

Americans with disabilities. Rackley (1994) studied self-efficacy among African American parents of children with disabilities and found that parents who were highly self-efficacious used more adaptive coping strategies than parents of children who were low in self-efficacy. In another study of parents of children with disabilities, Walker and Belgrave (1995) found self-efficacious beliefs to be associated with social support. In summary, the literature on self-efficacy suggests that self-efficacious beliefs can serve as a protective factor against stressors that might occur because of disability and/or ethnic minority status.

Thus, self-efficacy beliefs may be a useful intrapersonal resource for African Americans with chronic illnesses and disabilities. Take, for example, the situation of a person who has recently had a stroke with accompanying mobility limitations. Self-efficacious beliefs are likely to affect how much effort this individual puts into his or her physical therapy regimen and whether or not this individual adheres to other rehabilitation regimens. Under conditions where improvement in ability to walk does not occur as quickly as expected, this individual will likely persevere in physical therapy. Even when he or she experiences a setback, he or she is not likely to give up. Moreover, this individual is likely to maintain an optimistic outlook and to have positive emotional experiences. Consider another example of an individual who has had a job-related injury and is no longer able to go back to his or her preinjury employment. Under conditions of high self-efficacy, this individual is likely to continue his or her job-search efforts and maintain good spirits even if he or she experiences a long period of unemployment. Importantly, this individual is not likely to stop job-search efforts after being turned down for jobs. In fact, initial failure might reinforce the job-search efforts. Using these examples, it is not difficult to see how beneficial one's self-efficacious beliefs can be to one's functional outcomes and mental health status.

In spite of the beneficial aspects of having high self-efficacious beliefs, some research suggests that self-efficacy beliefs may be lower for members of ethnic minority groups than members of the majority culture (Hughes & Demo, 1989; Hunt & Hunt, 1977; Thompson & Spacapan, 1991). Lower self-efficacy among members of ethnic minority groups and members of disability group may be a realistic appraisal of social and economic conditions where there may be few opportunities for engaging in behaviors that lead to the execution of desired outcomes. For example, as noted in previous chapters, African Americans with disabilities and chronic illnesses have less access to medical and rehabilitation services than Whites. Consider the example of an African American who has had a stroke. This individual may not be able to participate in physical therapy because of access factors. We know that African Americans generally do not fare as well as Whites in the career and employment arenas because of a more disadvantaged position in this society. Thus, lower self-efficacious beliefs may reflect realistic appraisals of fewer opportunities.

The relationship between low self-efficacy beliefs and poor outcomes is cyclical. Low efficacy beliefs feed into the cycle of negativity where low effort leads to poor outcomes (i.e., no job)—which in turn reinforces low effort. The individual is caught up in a vicious cycle that is difficult to break out of. One way out is to strengthen one's self-efficacious beliefs while considering the socioenvironmental context of the person. (Strategies for increasing self-efficacy will be discussed in chapter 8.)

Other Aspects of Psychological Control

This discussion has shown that self-efficacy has several positive benefits on behavioral outcomes, as well as affective, emotional, and cognitive states. Self-efficacy is a type of psychological control that can be thought of as an intrapersonal resource. There are several other types of psychological control that are expected to contribute to the individual's ability to function competently. Locus of control is one such belief. Locus of control is a general orientation as to whether or not one believes that reinforcements for outcomes are due to internal factors or external factors (Rotter, 1966). Generally those individuals with an external locus of control orientation believe that outside factors such as luck or powerful others determine outcomes. Those with an internal locus of control orientation generally believe that they are responsible for the reward or punishments associated with their behaviors.

A person's locus of control orientation will determine his or her causal attribution for improvement or deterioration and subsequently whether or not he or she improves. For example, did I improve in my mobility following a stroke because I worked hard in physical therapy, or was it because of luck or fate? Having an internal locus of control orientation will most likely lead me to feel that if I participate in physical therapy, I will be rewarded by being able to walk again. Persons with an external locus of control orientation are more likely to feel that they do not have control over outcomes. Therefore I might be less likely to participate in physical therapy because I believe that my participation in physical therapy would not make a difference in my recovery. It is not difficult to see the similarities between having an internal locus of control orientation and high self-efficacy beliefs and an external locus of control orientation and low self-efficacy beliefs.

While an internal locus of control orientation is generally helpful, there are some conditions under which it may be maladaptive. These situations most often are those in which outcomes are objectively outside the person's control. Take, for example, the situation in which a person lives under conditions of extreme oppression and poverty. This individual could be highly motivated and may, in fact, work very hard, but environmental circumstances may prevent him from achieving his desired goals. Unfortunately this has been the plight for many African Americans, including African Americans with disabilities, who are caught in a cycle of poverty. Take another example of a wheelchair user who may be highly motivated to work but whose work site is architecturally inaccessible; no matter how motivated this individual is, she will not be able to work. An internal locus of control orientation, (i.e., assuming responsibility for poor outcomes) may, in fact, be maladaptive in this situation. When an individual takes responsibilities for something he or she cannot realistically control, he or she is likely to feel even worse in terms of self-concept. In this situation, it might be more adaptive for the individual to have an external locus of control orientation over this particular situation.

There are also health or medical situations in which an internal locus of control orientation is not adaptive. The experiences of some individuals with chronic illnesses provide an illustration. Under conditions of high chronicity, where illness symptoms may be uncontrollable or where disease progression is not controllable, an internal locus of control orientation may not be adaptive.

Burlew et al. (1995) studied a sample of 121 African Americans with sickle cell disease to determine the relationship between an internal locus of control orientation (along with other variables) and psychosocial adjustment (measured by anxiety and depression). Findings indicated that an internal health locus of control orientation was inversely related to anxiety. That is, persons who felt they had control over their health and associated outcomes were more anxious than those without this perception of internal control. The authors speculated that the episodic and unpredictable nature of sickle cell disease may offer an explanation for this inverse relationship. In the case of such a chronic illness as sickle cell disease, the belief and expectation that one has control may not be borne out in reality. People who expect to have control but do not may in fact become even more frustrated and anxious under conditions where there is little possibility for control.

Thus, the benefits of psychological control as an intrapersonal resource are situation specific. Many African Americans have functioned and currently function under conditions of little objective control. The institution of slavery, Jim Crow laws, and current levels of institutional discrimination in the employment and housing arenas provide examples of control of and power over African Americans by Whites in this country.

The implications of this are that African Americans should learn to recognize when internal control and high self-efficacy are and are not adaptive. This follows from an old AA prayer: "God, give me the strength to change the things I can, the courage to accept the things I cannot change, and the wisdom to know the difference."

COPING STRATEGIES

Coping strategies, as in the cases of self-efficacy and psychological control, are conceptualized in this chapter as interpersonal resources that can be used for maximizing adaptive functioning. *Coping* is defined as the process of managing external and internal demands that are appraised as exceeding the resources of the person. Coping consists of efforts, both action oriented and intrapsychic, used to manage, reduce, or minimize environmental and internal demands and conflicts (Lazarus & Folkman, 1984). Everyone uses coping strategies. Of relevance here is whether the coping strategies used are appropriate for helping the individual deal with a particular stressor. The question is what coping strategies are most effective for African Americans. Are some strategies more culturally congruent than others? These questions will be explored later in this chapter. First, an examination of coping will be provided.

There are two general types of coping: problem-focused coping and emotion-focused coping. Problem-focused coping involves efforts to remove or alter the source of stress. Emotion-focused coping efforts are directed at reducing the emotional distress brought on in a given situation (Carver, Scheier, & Weintraub, 1989). Some types of problem-focused coping strategies include (a) active coping (actually doing something to remove the stressor), (b) planning (thinking about how to cope with the stressor), and (c) seeking social support for emotional reasons (seeking advice and information). Examples of emotion-focused coping include (a) positive reinterpretation (viewing the stressor in a positive way), (b) denial (refusing to deal with the stressor), and (c) seeking social support for emotional reasons (seeking moral support, reassurance, affirmation). As noted earlier, problem-focused coping will work only if the individual has some control over the source of the problem. Therefore, there are some situations in which problem-focused coping is likely to be more adaptive and some situations in which emotion-focused coping is likely to be more adaptive.

An illustration of coping strategies can be shown by returning to the previous example of an individual who has recently had a stroke with accompanying mobility limitations. An individual who uses a problem-focused coping strategy might learn all he or she can about the stroke, engage in weekly physical therapy sessions, and plan how to use assistive devices. Under these conditions, the appraisal of the stroke as stressful would be reduced, and the functional ability (e.g., mobility) would most likely improve. This same example can be used to illustrate how emotion-focused coping could be used to deal with this stressor. This individual for example, might convince herself that mobility is not important and/or that the stroke has given a positive meaning to his or her life (positive reinterpretation).

While problem-focused coping may seem generally more adaptive, there are situations in which emotion-focused coping is better. For example, take a situation in which there is no realistic probability for improvement in a desired outcome (e.g., the person has had a spinal cord injury, and there is no medical reason to expect improved mobility). Problem-focused coping aimed at increasing mobility in this situation may in fact be distracting and unproductive. Under this condition, emotion-focused coping may be more effective. In this situation, if the person regulates his feelings and affective reactions to accept having a spinal cord injury, better adaptation would occur. As noted in a previous chapter, acceptance of one's disability and a positive attitude toward self facilitates adaptive functioning.

Surrounding oneself with people who provide emotional support that affirms the self is also an effective emotion-focused coping strategy. While problem-focused coping may not be adaptive if the aim is to change mobility status, it can be productive if the aim is to learn how to live with a mobility limitation. Under these conditions, the individual can obtain information, meet with similar others, and structure her external environment to support her mobility impairment. Emotion-focused coping seems to work better under conditions in which there may be little possibility of a change in long-term status.

The discussion of problem-focused versus emotion-focused coping highlights a critical difference between the two. In one case the person is doing something (i.e., being active), and in the other case the person is not. Examples can also be provided regarding the benefits of active versus passive coping strategies for adapting to a chronic illness or disability. Active coping is akin to problem-focused coping in the sense that the individual is actively doing something to change the situation. Engaging in physical therapy, exercising, educating oneself are all examples of active coping strategies. Passive coping strategies might involve denial, distraction (thinking about something else), and use of alcohol and drugs. While in general active coping strategies may seem more adaptive, there are circumstances in which passive coping strategies might be more adaptive. Doing nothing and denying the reality of a given situation may be the best strategy at the beginning of a traumatic event until the person can digest what has happened and until his or her condition has stabilized. Making decisions that may have long-term consequences may not be the best route to take at the beginning of a stressor. What is important to remember is that the effectiveness of a particular coping strategy is situation specific, with some coping strategies more beneficial in some situations and others more beneficial in others.

Culturally, African Americans may be more likely to use emotion-focused and passive coping strategies relative to Whites. As discussed in chapter 3, spirituality and the value of turning a negative into a positive support the strategies of using positive reinterpretation and finding meaning and purpose to both positive and negative situations. These are two emotion-focused coping strategies. However, African Americans have also learned to work hard and to provide support to each other—problem-solving and active coping strategies. Of relevance here is for African Americans to be flexible and use the coping strategy that is most beneficial. (Some of these strategies are discussed in chapter 8.)

RESEARCH ON COPING AND ADJUSTMENT AMONG AFRICAN AMERICANS

Several studies have focused on coping strategies and other cognitive behavioral factors as they relate to adaptive functioning among individuals with disabilities and chronic illness. Some of the research has been conducted by the author and others on African Americans with sickle cell disease.

Belgrave and Washington (1986) found among adolescents with sickle cell disease that an assertive coping style was linked to their ability to manage painful episodes. Adolescents reported less disruption in activities of daily living when having a painful episode if they had an assertive coping style. This assertive coping style is an active, problem-focused way of dealing with painful sickle cell disease episodes. Adolescents in our study who were able to make requests and to inform others of their needs within the home, school, peer, and community domains fared better.

Gil, Williams, Thompson, and Kinney (1991) found that among patients with sickle cell disease, negative thinking and passive adherence were associated with more severe pain, less activity, and distress. These passive coping strategies were also associated with more health care services utilization. The results of this study suggest that passive adherence to prescribed treatments and rehabilitation regiments is not always good. The person should assume some degree of control over his or her treatment. Control over treatment within the medical and rehabilitation environment is likely to be especially difficult for some African Americans, who may feel intimidated by higher-status professionals. However, these skills can be learned, and strategies for gaining these skills will be discussed in chapter 8.

Tyler (1978) has conceptualized active coping somewhat differently than Lazarus and Folkman (1984) and Carver, Scheier, and Weintraub (1989). Tyler's conceptualization of coping is also useful when thinking of active coping as an intrapersonal resource for African Americans with chronic illnesses and disabilities, and this conceptualization also lends itself nicely to identifying strategies for enhancing adaptive coping.

Active coping, as conceptualized by Tyler (1978), is a cognitive behavioral factor that impacts how an individual functions. According to Tyler, active coping is the way an individual copes with both adverse and favorable conditions: it involves his or her initiative, goal setting, planning, and the effort made to attain goals. An individual who actively copes effectively takes responsibilities for what happens to him or her and actively plans for and carries out behaviors to enhance his or her well-being. Using this definition of active coping, one can see how closely it is akin to the concepts of self-efficacy and psychological control. One can also see how active coping can help one achieve empowerment.

The beneficial effect of coping on adjustment to disability has been demonstrated in several studies (Affleck, Urrows, Tennen, & Higgins, 1992; Brown, Doepke, & Kaslow, 1993; Hanson, Buckelew, Hewett, & O'Neal, 1993; Zea, Belgrave, Townsend, Jarama, & Banks, 1996). In a study of African American and Latinos with disabilities, Zea et al. (1996) found that active coping was a significant predictor of psychological adjustment (i.e., depression) among African Americans and Latinos with disabilities. Persons who scored higher on an active coping scale were less depressed. This finding underscores the value of active coping in improving one's mental health and affective states.

In summary, given that self-efficacious beliefs have positive effects in the emotional, cognitive, and behavioral domains, programs to increase these beliefs are worthy of investigation. Persons who are high in self-efficacy (as compared to low in self-efficacy) try harder, are not as despondent when they fail, and are more likely to succeed eventually.

It is important to remind the reader that self-efficacious beliefs that emphasize individual achievement of goals should be integrated with collective efficacy. Communal and interdependent orientations of African Americans support the attainment of group goals along with individual goals. The West African proverb "I am because we are, and we are because I am" implies that people of African descent and people with disabilities will all do well or will all do poorly. This belief suggests that one contributes to and gains from similar others. Therefore, as will be seen in chapters 7 and 8, the author recommends access to and involvement with a group of similar others in the attainment of goals.

When social and environmental conditions are oppressive, as may be the case when discrimination, poverty, racism, and limited employment opportunities exist, active coping can help the individual overcome barriers and function more effectively. For African Americans with disabilities, strategies to enhance active coping may be beneficial.

As noted, active coping and self-efficacy are related to each other. Persons who use active coping and problem-solving coping strategies are more likely to have high self-efficacy about their ability to achieve a desired outcome. These two constructs are also related to social support. The overlap among these constructs has implications for understanding the mechanisms through which self-efficacy, active coping, and social support influence outcomes such as mental health and employment. Furthermore, these concepts can be used to provide a framework for developing programs to improve outcomes for African Americans with chronic illnesses and disabilities.

THE RELATIONSHIPS AMONG ACTIVE COPING, SELF-EFFICACY, PSYCHOLOGICAL CONTROL, AND SOCIAL SUPPORT

Throughout this chapter, it has been made salient that social support can be used as a coping strategy. According to Carver, Scheier, and Weintraub (1989), material, informational, and emotional support are specific coping strategies that people may use to cope with stressors. We saw in the last chapter how social support helps to decrease poor mental health and to increase adaptive functioning. Moreover, our work has shown that social support from families, kin, and informal resources to be especially helpful for African Americans. Social support, then, can be a means through which self-efficacious beliefs and active coping are achieved.

Let's return again to the example of a person who has had a stroke. One way in which this person could cope might be to seek out informational support from a health care provider regarding the prognosis and recommended treatment for his or her condition. Another person might need financial or material support and may ask a friend to loan him or her his car to go to a medical appointment or to borrow money to purchase medication (material support). Another way to cope might be by joining a support group of stroke survivors. Here the group may provide the person with comfort, reassurance, warmth, and positive self-regard that can strengthen his/her ability to cope with adversity.

What is important to note here is that individuals who cope more effectively seem to know how to seek out and access the appropriate types of and forms of support. Providing people with skills for identifying and accessing support is discussed in the next chapter. The source and type of support should be culturally congruent with the worldview and beliefs of African Americans.

Self-efficacy is also related to social support. Individuals who are high in self-efficacy are likely to have environmental social supports that are reinforcing and culturally congruent. For persons with chronic illnesses and disabilities, the development of efficacious beliefs within a framework of supportive others who provide information to each other and who learn skills from each other is important.

SUMMARY

Using active coping strategies and learning how to access and give social support in a culturally congruent manner can be empowering for African Americans with chronic illnesses and disabilities. In this context, African Americans with disabilities and chronic illnesses can help each other to achieve their desired goals. Once these intrapersonal resources are developed within an individual, family, or community, they become powerful resources. These resources do not cost money. They can be obtained by the powerless and the disenfranchised. They can make a difference in the quality of life for African Americans with disabilities.

PART III

Culturally Congruent Approaches

7

Guidelines for Implementing a Social Support Intervention

As discussed in chapter 5, social support serves as a buffer against stress and other aversive conditions African Americans with disabilities and chronic illnesses might face. Under stressful conditions, individuals with social support will have better outcomes than those without. Therefore, programs which teach individuals to identify, access, and use supportive relationships may be beneficial. This is the focus of this chapter.

Social support groups are natural and culturally congruent systems for African Americans. These groups can build upon the strengths of traditional family, friend, kin, religious, and community networks. As discussed in chapter 3, values that are communal, relationship- and interpersonally oriented encourage the use of a group of similar others for

The author acknowledges the contributions of all individuals who have collaborated with her in conducting social support interventions: Dr. Sylvia Walker of Howard University; Sonia Banks and Lisbeth Jarama of The George Washington University; Cynthia Burley, Milagros McGuire, Joan Wills, Ruth Royal Hill, Mary Ann Mesmer, and Alturo Rodriguis of RSA. Finally, and most importantly, appreciation is extended to all consumers with disabilities who have been members of our groups.

Some of the guidelines offered in this chapter were adapted from a manual titled "Enhancing Outcomes Among African Americans and Latinos with Disabilities Through Empowerment and Support." Faye Z. Belgrave, Maria C. Zea, Sylvia Walker, Sonia R. Banks, S. Lisbeth Jarama, and Tiffany Townsend (authors). The manual is available from the first author at the Department of Psychology, Virginia Commonwealth University, Richmond, Va.

Table 7.1
Steps to Implementing a Social Support Group Intervention

- Clarify the purpose of the program, its objectives, and desired outcomes.
- Define group structure.
- Develop and implement a plan for recruiting and retaining participants.
- Develop and implement program content.

addressing problems and concerns. Social support groups can be a medium through which individuals solve immediate problems and learn how to access and use existing social networks for addressing future problems.

Guidelines for implementing a social support group intervention are provided in this chapter. The author and colleagues have developed, implemented, and evaluated several support group interventions with African Americans and other ethnic minority groups with disabilities, and much of what is presented in this chapter is based on the experiences of these observers who have worked with support groups. While the author's interventions have been geared toward groups of working-age African Americans and Latinos with disabilities, the guidelines provided in this chapter should be useful to individuals from other groups.

An intervention program starts with a goal, purpose, or objective. These must be shared among group members. The structure and format of the group must also be well defined prior to the start of the sessions in order for the groups to be efficient and effective. Recruitment and retention of group members is an important activity—no matter how well developed a program is, it will not be successful unless members attend sessions. Finally, the content of the sessions, or what is actually discussed and accomplished in the sessions, must be developed and implemented in a sequential manner. The content of a social support intervention should contain activities and exercises that teach members how to identify, access, and use supportive network members, organizations, and agencies. Activities should be tied to desired outcomes (i.e., increased employment, more positive attitudes, better mental health, etc.). The steps to implementing a social support intervention are discussed in this chapter (see Table 7.1).

DEFINING THE OBJECTIVES OF THE GROUP

The first step is to identify the desired outcomes of the social support intervention. These outcomes should be consistent with the wishes of group members. There should be congruence between leaders/sponsors and group members as to what these outcomes are. For example, in one of our groups, we (as mental health professionals) were interested in improved mental health (i.e., increased self-esteem, decreased depression, etc.). However, participants (consumers with disabilities) were more interested in employment, housing, and other more immediate basic concerns. The desired outcomes will define the structure and content of group activities. The objectives of our social support intervention were to improve outcomes of African Americans with disabilities across several dimensions, including employment, mental health, and functioning in activities of daily living. As noted in previous chapters, employment was considered an important outcome because of its centrality to quality of life for U.S. citizens. Work (or lack of) in this country often defines how a person views him- or herself and how this person is seen by others. Under conditions where there are limited power and resources, employment becomes a mechanism for gaining equity. Among African Americans with disabilities, the vast majority are not employed (only 16% are employed) (Bowe, 1991). These individuals subsequently face problems in related areas, including substandard housing, low levels of education, and inadequate medical care and rehabilitative services. We wanted members to obtain jobs and to change their attitudes and beliefs about their ability to find and maintain employment.

Persons with disabilities may also be at increased risk for poor mental health outcomes because of stressors related to unemployment, ethnic minority, and disability status. Therefore, improved mental health outcomes such as decreased stress and depression are also important for this population. Depression and stress interfere with one's ability to function in every domain, including the work domain. We wanted our participants to improve their self-esteem and confidence in themselves individually and as African Americans and people with disabilities. Therefore, another outcome was improved self attitudes and attitudes toward persons with disabilities. We wanted participants to learn how to cope with stress and adversity within the supportive environment of our group and to extend what they learned within the group to situations outside the support group environment.

We also desired improvements in functioning in activities of daily living in the home, in the church, and in the community. Isolation may be a problem, and people with disabilities may become isolated because of physical limitations and/or stigmatizing attitudes from others. Therefore, routine activities such as attending church, taking care of a relative, and shopping may be neglected. It is important to emphasize again that the goals and objectives must be shared by group members and facilitators.

Once the objectives of the group have been clearly defined, aspects of group structure must be defined. These must be done in a manner that is culturally congruent and conducive to the group meeting its goals.

GROUP STRUCTURE

Several aspects of group structure should be considered before sessions begin. These include (1) group composition, (2) leadership, (3) responsibility of leaders and participants, (4) group norms, (5) size of group, (6) environment or setting, (7) duration of sessions, and (8) presentation of materials.

Group Composition

The intervention may not be beneficial for everyone, and some individuals may benefit more than others. Participants of our group sessions were consumers of Rehabilitation Services Administration (RSA), a state rehabilitation agency. The criteria for participation in our program was developed in consultation with officials and rehabilitation specialists at RSA. Participants in our groups were fairly new to the agency (i.e., had been clients of the agency for less than three or four months). We also thought, because of the intense level of involvement expected from participants, that the program would be more beneficial to those who were not involved in any other training activities. Participants had to be motivated and willing to change and be able to attend sessions on a weekly basis. Finally we wanted members who could contribute to group discussion and activities. Therefore one criterion for inclusion was that the group member be able to communicate with other group members. In situations where one's disability may limit certain types of communication, mechanisms should be put in place so that all members can communicate with each other. Interpreters will be necessary for heterogeneous groups of deaf and hearing participants. Individuals experiencing severe emotional disturbances (i.e., exhibiting psychotic and/or delusional thinking, suicidal, and/or aggressive acting-out behaviors will probably not benefit and should not be included in this type of group). Individuals with severe levels of mental retardation (defined as substantially below average intelligence with severe deficits in behaviors) are also unlikely to benefit.

Depending upon the objectives of the program, homogeneous groups of individuals with similar disabilities may be more effective. For example, the needs of a group of individuals who are disabled because of addiction may differ from that of a group of individuals who are disabled because of kidney disease. However, we found that although our groups were diverse in disability type, they were able to meet their goals collectively. The types of disabilities of participants in our group included seizure disorders, neurological impairments, physical disabilities, cognitive impairments, mental illness, and drug addiction. Members were also diverse by nature of socioeconomic conditions, age, and gender. Participants had the commonalities of being African American, consumers of RSA, of working age (primarily under 55), and unemployed at the time of initiation. All participants also had the potential to become employable. In spite of diverse backgrounds, group members came together and worked cohesively as a group.

Leadership

Group leadership is an important aspect of group structure that should be given serious consideration. Leaders provide information and resources, direct the group toward accomplishing its objectives, and serve as influential models. In general, our efforts support the recommendation that the leader be similar to group participants in relevant aspects. Similar others are powerful motivators for change. Within a social support group, the group members may better relate to a similar rather than a dissimilar other. Subsequently, group members are more likely to model desired behavior and engage in suggested behavioral change activities. From this perspective, the leader should be an African American with a disability.

The selection of the leader will depend on the type of group, the characteristics of group participants, and the needs of the group. For example, our groups consisted of African Americans with different types of disabilities. Therefore, our peer leader was an African American consumer of RSA with a disability. If the group consists of a singular disability group, a member of that group should be selected for leadership. If the group members consist of all males, a male leader would probably be more effective than a female leader.

When groups need a professional or technical expert that is not available among group members, a coleadership model may be used by having both peer and professional leaders. In our groups, both professionals and peer leaders have been used. These leaders served complementary roles with each supporting different types of activities.

The role of the leader should be clear. In our groups, we have used the term *facilitator* rather than leader. The term *leader* implies that the person is in charge and has the major influence in the group. A facilitator, in contrast, advises and directs the activities of the group and works on behalf of group members.

Responsibilities of Group Members

Introductory sessions should be devoted to making sure participants understand their responsibilities in the group. In keeping with the collectivist orientation of African Americans and the nature of a support group intervention, it is important that group members understand that they are responsible for individually and collectively meeting the group's goals. Members are responsible for each other's accomplishments as well as each other's failures. With this orientation, the joy of one member obtaining employment is shared by all members. The disappointment of one member not getting a desired job is experienced within the supportive environment of the group.

The following are suggested responsibilities to convey to group participants. In our groups, members were responsible for:

1. attending all meetings on time;
2. participating in discussions and group activities;
3. sharing resources and information with other group members;
4. being flexible and willing to change; and
5. respecting other group members at all times.

In addition to adhering to the responsibilities of group members, group leaders (facilitators) have additional responsibilities. These may include:

1. structuring the activities of the group so that the group can meet its objectives;
2. encouraging interaction among group members and seeing that all members are actively involved in discussions and exercises;
3. assisting in obtaining any needed resources for the group;
4. clarifying and interpreting information for group members.

We have found that it is important for the facilitators to understand that it is not their responsibility to lecture at or tell participants what to do, but to serve as an advisor. Because the focus of the intervention is on participants learning how to access and use supportive networks to address their own problems, the leader can model these skills within the group. Within this context, the group is a laboratory in which members can practice activities and learn new skills and techniques. It is helpful to have training sessions for group leaders or facilitators so that they understand how they are to function within the group. In cases where the group facilitators are professionals, whose normal activities may be to direct and negotiate on behalf of clients, they must understand their role in the social support group is different. In one support group led by a rehabilitation specialist, group members rejected a directive leader who insisted on calling the shots and telling everyone what to do.

Group Norms

During the normal process of group formation, norms will develop. Norms are acceptable ways of behaving in groups and help the group to move along and meet its goals and objectives. Norms may be stated or implicit (not stated). Without norms, the group cannot function effectively because there would be no commonly acceptable ways of behaving. Although the group leader can suggest some norms, it is important that group members develop their own norms to govern their behavior while within the group. While norms may develop naturally over time, given that most groups will be time limited, it may be helpful to have group members articulate norms during the first few sessions. In our groups, some of the articulated norms were:

1. being respectful to each other and not using profanity;
2. not talking about confidential information provided by other group members outside the group;
3. greeting one another when entering the group;
4. saying a prayer at the start of each session;
5. not smoking; and
6. working together as a group.

While some of the norms were quite general (i.e., working together as a group), others were quite specific (i.e., not smoking). The importance of spirituality in our group was reflected by the decision of group members to say a prayer at the beginning of each session.

The articulation of norms early on serves several purposes. First, as noted, group norms regulate behaviors of group members so that groups can meet their goals and objectives. Second, cohesiveness and solidarity of the group are strengthened through the identification of shared ways of behaving. Third, the norms reinforce the similarity of values among group members.

Group Size

The group should be small enough that group members can interact with each other easily and everyone can be involved in the discussion. However, the group should not be too small because the potential resourcefulness of group members will be lost if there are too few group members. In general, a group with only three or four members will not be as resourceful as a larger group. Groups of 8 to 12 individuals seem best for this purpose. The group leader(s) adds an additional one or two members to the group.

It may also be useful to pair group members two by two, as "buddies" with each other. These members may be in touch with each other between sessions and serve additional supportive functions for each other. Buddies may call each other or get together to work on homework assignments or other out of class activities. Members can also be encouraged to call or contact members other than buddies if desired.

Environment/Setting

The social support sessions should be held within a convenient and accessible environment. Facilities such as community centers, churches, and a multipurpose room in a housing development may be used. Settings within the community serve practical functions. When a program is focused on teaching persons how to identify, access, and use supportive networks, the community is a natural setting in which to begin practicing acquired skills.

Locating one's program within a community is congruent culturally insofar as African Americans are more likely to be comfortable and productive in settings that reflect their everyday reality. We used community-based social service agencies for our group meetings. Our participants were familiar with these agencies and had used them prior to the intervention. Facilities should be located in places that are accessible. We found participants were more likely to attend meetings at facilities within rather than outside their communities. For persons with disabilities, accessibility both to and within the facility is necessary. Easy and affordable access to public transportation is critical. Lack of transportation has been identified as a major barrier to employment for African Americans with disabilities (Belgrave & Walker, 1991a).

The facility should be accessible once the person arrives at the facility. The meeting room(s) should be pleasant, well-lit, and large enough to accommodate the group members with space for breaking up for smaller group activities (an additional room may be used). The room should also be large enough to accommodate wheelchair users and members with assistive devices. A circular or rectangular table can be used to facilitate discussions and interactive activities. A flip chart or blackboard is helpful to highlight important points made during the discussions.

In our groups, we found it helped to serve refreshments. The availability of refreshments facilitated discussions during the more informal premeeting part of the sessions. Participants would often arrive early to the sessions and informally chat over refreshments as they waited for the session to begin.

Duration of Sessions

Sessions should ideally meet once a week for two to three hours for 8 to 12 weeks. Although we have run groups for only seven weeks, members have consistently requested that the number of sessions be extended. Alternatively, members may decide to spread meetings over several months.

The natural formation of the group will take about two to three sessions. During these first few sessions, a major task is for individual members to come together to function collectively as a group. By the fourth week, the group should function as a cohesive unit. At this time, the major activity of the group will be to focus on meeting the group's objectives. The group will need an additional three or four sessions to internalize information, practice new skills, begin to change attitudes, and find new ways of approaching problems.

Presentation of Materials

All written and verbal information should be presented in a manner that is clear and easy for the members to understand. It is the facilitators' responsibility to make sure they (or other group members) do not become too esoteric or academic. Communication should be understandable to all members.

Use of both verbal and written forms of communication is encouraged. Written materials should be discussed orally, and participants should be encouraged to reinterpret and relate information to their own experiences. Members can be encouraged to write important points on a board or in a place where they can be seen.

Members should be encouraged to jot down ideas and keep a written journal of what happens in the group. It is also helpful to have each group member keep a log or a journal of relevant activities and events that may occur outside the group. The journal might include notations of their feelings about certain activities, progress they have made in accomplishing their goals, and their evaluation of the group process. If one of the group objectives is to find employment, an employment log of activities directed at seeking employment, outcomes, and reactions to efforts should be useful.

RECRUITMENT AND RETENTION: HOW TO RECRUIT MEMBERS AND KEEP THEM INTERESTED

Once the objectives of the group and aspects of structure are clear, the next task is to recruit members into the group. Recruitment may be done by consumer groups, by rehabilitation professionals, or other organized groups and persons.

Establishing Collaborative Relationships

The first step is to obtain the support of the sponsoring organization, consumer group, or agencies from which people will be recruited. Several meetings may be needed to inform potential collaborators of the program's objectives and activities. If you are not a member of the organization or group, this is a time to learn more about it. We targeted consumers of Rehabilitation Service Administration, the state rehabilitation agency, as our participants. Therefore, initial meetings were held with officials and counselors at RSA to discuss our program and learn more about consumers of RSA. The commitment and support of key individuals at an early stage is critical to the success of recruitment efforts. Consumers should also be involved in the recruitment process early on. For example, through consumers we learned the importance of holding sessions within the communities where individuals reside. If there is no organized consumer group, the rehabilitation specialist (or a staff person) can recommend consumers to serve as advisors to the program staff. For our groups, RSA referred peer facilitators who were consumers of RSA. These individuals then became program staff, with responsibilities comparable to the professional facilitator.

Recruiting Participants into the Program

Once key persons within an agency and organization are involved and committed to see the program succeed, the next step is to distribute information about the program to potential participants. We designed a flyer that provided information on what (purpose of program), when (sequencing of program), how (methods to be used in program), and where (meeting place). The overall objective of the program was stated as a program to help RSA consumers learn skills and techniques to help themselves. These flyers were given to rehabilitation personnel to distribute to their clients.

If a person was interested in learning more about the program, he or she completed a referral form that provided us with his or her name, phone number, and the best times to call. Each person was contacted within a few days of this referral. It is important not to wait too long following the initial referral, so that the potential participant's interest will not be lost. In cases were the person does not have a telephone, identifying a person within the agency or organization to serve as a point of contact is helpful. Expect that some of the participants will not have telephones.

The initial phone call should provide potential participants with additional information about the program and the opportunity to answer any questions he or she might have. More specific information about the time and place of the sessions may also be provided during this call. Typically consumers will want to know what they can get out of the program, (i.e., will it help them to find a job?, a place to live?, etc.). Consumers may also want specific information on the whereabouts of the program.

Prospective group members should be mailed a confirmation letter about a week before the sessions start. This letter confirms the specifics outlined in the phone call. Participants are asked to notify project staff if they cannot attend the first (or subsequent) session(s).

Retention

Once participants have been recruited into the group, efforts must be made to maintain initial levels of enthusiasm and retain participants. During the first session, the expectations of group members should be addressed. For example, during our first session, some members had come believing the program would find them jobs. Here, it was important for participants to understand our program was not a job-search service, but a support group that would help them to develop the skills and access the resources they could then use to find employment. If members' expectations are not addressed early and specifically, disillusion and disappointments are likely to undermine their (and others) progress in the group. In cases where there is no compromise regarding group expectations, it may be better for the member to leave the group.

Several strategies can be used to maintain high levels of group participation. Buddies can call each other during the week and, in doing so, provide encouragement, support, and information to each other. Weekly reminder phone calls from project staff and organizers also help, especially in the initial stages. The peer facilitators made these calls for our groups.

Participant incentives may also encourage regular attendance. In our groups, participants were given certificates if they attended all or most sessions. These certificates were appreciated by members and viewed as a symbol of their accomplishments. Some participants also used them in their job-search efforts to demonstrate to potential employers they had participated in a program designed to enhance their skills.

If funding is available, monetary incentives also help in recruiting and retaining participants. Most of our participants were unemployed, with limited financial resources. Therefore, monetary incentives were good motivators.

However, if there are no monetary incentives, support group developers should not be discouraged. As noted, nonmonetary incentives, such as certificates, awards, and special recognition, are good motivators. Importantly, once members have attended a few sessions, the sessions become the motivator. Members want to attend as they develop new relationships and learn how to access existing supportive relationships within their community.

CONTENT OF SOCIAL SUPPORT SESSIONS

The description of content in this chapter relies heavily upon the author's experience in social support groups convened. Exercises and activities that seemed to work in the groups she and colleagues convened are provided. Consistent with the theme of this chapter, sessions were generally oriented toward teaching members to identify and access social support appropriately. The sessions also focused on how to be a good provider of support. In essence, the group provided a medium in which activities could be carried out and skills could be developed through practice, feedback, and critique among group members.

Since a desired group outcome was employment, many of the activities were directed at helping participants develop skills and identify resources to find employment. While the temporal sequencing of sessions and activities are not fixed, activities were generally designed to build upon what was developed earlier. An outline of the objectives and illustrative activities and exercises are discussed for seven sessions.

Session One: Program Introduction (What Is This Program All About?)

The objective of the first session was to introduce the program and explain the program objectives. The format and structure (participatory nature of group, meeting schedule, responsibilities of group members) should be discussed at this first session. This is also the time to answer any questions and address participants' expectations. It is important that members are clear as to what they can expect to obtain by participating in the group in order to prevent later feelings of disillusionment over unmet expectations.

An icebreaker exercise can be used to get members talking and to give them an opportunity to get to know one another. The icebreaker exercise we used was to have each member say his or her name and tell the group two reasons for participating in the program. Members were also asked to say the name of the previous individual who spoke and that person's reasons for being at the session. If data are to be collected for evaluation purposes, it should be done at this first session, preferably at the beginning.

Session Two: Developing Group Cohesiveness and Identifying a Social Support Network (Who Is There to Help Me?)

The first exercise can be an icebreaker exercise whereby members continue to develop rapport and learn about fellow group members. In our sessions, we asked members to introduce themselves and tell about a supportive activity they had performed for another person and one that had been performed for them.

A suggested second exercise is to begin to develop group norms. As noted previously, norms are important insofar as they help regulate the behavior of group members and help the group achieve its goals. By discussing and coming to a consensus about what will govern group interactions, members began to make a commitment to the group and to take responsibility for the group's activities.

Our third activity was designed to get members to start to thinking about providers of support and members of their supportive network. In our group, we introduced the concept of a supportive network by asking members to think about what the word *net* meant. Members came up with several suggestions (e.g., provides a way to catch things, used to catch fish, provides a place to sleep if you tie the net between two trees, holds things in place, etc.).

Once members understood what the word *network* meant, they drew a "network circle." This provided a visual representation of each member's social support network. This circle may include one's family, friends, neighbors, ex-coworkers, organizations, agencies, or any other supportive person or resource the member can think of. We also asked members to draw themselves in the middle of the circle and to place within the circle the other persons at distances to represent the varying levels of distance and closeness they feel with the person (or organization).

Once members complete their network circle, engage them in a discussion of their networks. The following topics can be discussed: Why are certain people at various points on the circle? What role do members play in accessing their network? Are there people in the network who are not called upon to provide support? Whom do members provide support to?

The final activity of this session can be a buddy matching activity. This activity can be introduced as a way to add another person to their network circle. Buddies are asked to share information about themselves and are encouraged to exchange telephone numbers.

Session Three: Types of Social Support (How Do I Distinguish Types of Support and Link These Types with Network Members?)

By the third session, members may understand that the group members, in effect, provide support to each other. During this session, members will learn to identify different types of support and who the most appropriate provider is for a particular type of support. A first exercise may have members discuss a situation in which they needed or sought support from someone in their network over the previous week. Each situation can be discussed in terms of whom they called upon (i.e., brother, spouse, friend, social services), what specific help was needed (type of support), and what the outcome was (support provided, not provided). Ask members to say how they felt when they asked for and received the help. In this session, it may be helpful to acknowledge that sometimes asking for help evokes shame or anger or other negative emotions from the recipient. These feelings must be dealt with. The facilitator may discuss ways of handling these negative emotions. For example, when there is reciprocation, negative feelings are more likely to be replaced with self-fulling ones. One outcome from this exercise was that group members began to connect with one another as they shared common reactions to asking for and receiving help.

The goal of the second exercise was for members to understand the different types of support and how a particular type of support can be linked to a specific need. The categories of emotional, informational, and material types of support provided good distinctions (see chapter 5). Emotional support can be defined as being listened to, receiving encouragement and praise, and feeling loved and cared for. Informational support can be defined as receiving information or learning something, acquiring knowledge and advice. Material support can be defined as receiving something tangible, such as money, transportation, or help with child-care. Participants can demonstrate their understanding of different types of support by giving examples of different types of support. The facilitators may provide examples: sharing a job lead (informational support), writing a letter (material support), and getting encouragement (emotional support). When participants have a clear understanding of the types of support, the next exercise can be done to gain a further understanding of how to access the appropriate type of support. Persons may work with their buddies for this exercise.

Situations in which support is needed can be generated by each pair. These members can then discuss the appropriate type of support and who might be the most appropriate provider of this type of support. Members can complete a chart with three columns: (a) the situation where support is needed, (b) the type of support, and (c) the most appropriate source and provider of support.

A group discussion following this exercise should emphasize the importance of matching the different types of support with the source. For example, an employment counselor may not be the most appropriate person to ask for help with baby-sitting. A friend or neighbor might be more appropriate. If you are feeling depressed and lonely and need someone to talk to, your mother may be the most appropriate source for this type of support. However, if your mother has not been able to help you in the past, consider someone else in your network.

Another exercise we used allowed members to apply what has been learned to employment efforts. In a group discussion, members are asked to share their techniques and resources for finding employment. A list can be developed. This provides members with an opportunity to be supportive to each other by sharing any resources or job leads they might have.

Members can review their social support networks and determine what support is available to assist them in securing employment. For example, one member of the group might have a relative who works in an industry desired by another group member. Another might realize he or she can give his or her neighbors his or her resume, and so on.

Group members and facilitators can also provide information on what resources are available to the general public, (i.e., employment bulletins, community bulletin board, telephone job lines, job training centers, etc.).

Session Four: Learning to Be Supportive (How Do I Give Support?)

In this session, participants learn how to attend to the needs of others and how to give appropriate types of support. A key assumption underlying this exercise is that in order to receive support one must be a provider of support.

A good start-up exercise is to have each member discuss an experience of being supportive to persons within and outside their networks. The discussion should be directed at discussing how members feel when they give support. For example, members might report feeling joy or satisfaction that they are building a relationship, fulfilling a spiritual mission, and so on. This exercise ties into the one in the previous session whereby members discussed how they felt when they received support. Members should also be directed to discuss when they are likely to give support and the types of support they are good at giving. For example, if a member is good with children, he or she may want to offer child-care support. A person who knows the public transportation system in the city well may want to be a guide for a person who is less adept with the public transportation system.

A discussion of volunteering may also be relevant during this session.

Members can discuss causes they endorse and be encouraged to volunteer for such causes if they have time. In addition to the positive feeling volunteering brings, volunteer work may lead to the development of new skills that can be transferred to the job market.

The group can engage in a discussion of how being an effective provider of support means being aware of the needs of the individual and being able to match the needs with the appropriate type or provider of support. If one cannot provide what is needed, referring the person to another resource can be a form of support. A second exercise provided members with the opportunity to provide emotional support by role playing how to be an effective (active) listener. The facilitator can list on the board active listening behaviors. These include body posture oriented toward speaker, eye contact with speaker, and acknowledging the speaker's comments. The active listener acknowledges that he or she understands what is being said by restating essential points and confirms that the person is finished talking by asking if he or she has more to say. Members can practice active listening in a supportive relationship through role play. Two group members can practice speaking and active listening in front of the group. The group provides feedback regarding whether or not the listener has been responsive to the speaker through his or her body language and verbal behaviors.

Another exercise can be directed at providing informational support through job interview practice for groups in which employment is desired. Members can role play job interview scenarios, with members switching the interviewer and interviewee roles. Group members can provide feedback on role players' verbal and nonverbal behaviors. A homework assignment may be to have members identify an agency or organization or persons they would like to do volunteer work with.

Session Five: Empowerment Versus Dependence (I Can Versus I Don't Think I Can).

The objective of this session is for participants to understand that their network and supportive relationships can be a source of empowerment for them. Another objective is for participants to understand they can empower themselves through the acquisition of skills and knowledge that may be accessed through their network. Additional activities directed toward empowerment are reviewed in chapter 8.

An initial exercise can be a discussion of what empowerment means and how people empower themselves. For example, empowerment occurs when one learns a skill or picks up a tool that helps to accomplish goals. For example, if I ask someone to teach me how to fill out an application, I empower myself to learn how to apply for a job. If I ask a friend to take a computer course with me, we empower each other by motivating each other to learn a new skill. Positive self attitudes are also empowering. Efforts directed at increasing one's self-esteem, one's ability to relate to others, and one's confidence will be rewarded by more purposeful action.

The next activity can be directed at getting participants to understand how one's network can be used as an empowerment tool. Members can list ways in which they can empower themselves either by giving or receiving support from their network. A related exercise could have members list ways in which employment goals can be reached by using their network. For example, one member may have a personal contact at a firm that another individual is interested in.

A discussion of disempowerment may also be helpful. For example, we disempower ourselves if we become overly dependent on specific persons within our network and do not rely upon our own resources to accomplish a task.

In another exercise, members might discuss how to meet goals by developing appropriate support-seeking skills. Scenarios can be presented by the facilitators or group members and then discussed in the group.

A final suggested exercise is to have participants begin to track their employment efforts by keeping a daily journal. This journal will provide each member with feedback about daily efforts to utilize resources within and outside their network to find employment. The journal should report the date, the time, the activity, and what was actually done.

Session Six: Cultural Aspects (What Values Are Important to Me and My Community?)

In this session, group members learn how cultural values can facilitate or inhibit desired goals. In our groups, members also discussed what values are common to African Americans and how these might differ from the values of other ethnic groups. Values were discussed within the context of social support. For example, is it easier for African Americans to give and receive support from kin and family than other ethnic groups because of the African American extended family?

An initial activity may be to discuss core cultural values among African Americans. Culture is defined as shared ways of thinking and behaving among a group of people. A review of chapter 3, which focuses on African American values, may be helpful for this task. Members should be asked to come up with their own values before they are provided by the facilitator.

A discussion of how relationships may differ among African Americans and other ethnic groups may serve as a further illustration of core African American values. This discussion may include a discussion of the central role that the family, including the extended family, plays in the lives of African Americans. Participants may provide examples from their own experiences of what their family means to them.

Spirituality as a source of support may also be discussed during this session. In our group, members spoke of the importance of attending church, praying, and other religious and spiritual practices.

In our groups, members got into small groups and discussed their perception of positive and negative aspects of social support within the African American community. For example, African Americans may have a greater willingness to look out for and take care of less fortunate family members (positive outcome). However, when this fosters over-dependency, it can sometimes lead to strained relationships for both the recipient and the provider.

A discussion of how being African American affects employment opportunities may also be helpful during this session. For example, some participants in our groups felt African Americans were at a disadvantage in the employment arena because of racism and discrimination. However, other participants felt that because African Americans are flexible, they can adapt to whatever situation. It may be useful for the facilitator to acknowledge discrimination based on ethnicity and disability, but to redirect the participant to think about how he or she can empower him or herself. A related activity is to have group members identify those aspects of the African American culture that may help or hinder their opportunities to find a job. For example, African Americans may use time differently from White Americans. The phrase "CP," or colored people's, time may be a cultural norm. However, lack of attention to present time may cause the person to lose the job if he or she does not show up for an interview on time. Likewise, if the job requirements call for independent work, an interpersonal or communal orientation may not be adaptive in this environment. In these situations, the employee must be sensitive to the requirements of the job and adjust his or her behavior accordingly. Beliefs in spirituality and the faith that this belief brings may reduce the stress associated with finding employment and enable the person to cope with unemployment.

A final activity for this session may be to have group members affirm themselves culturally by focusing on the strengths of the African American community. Since some of our sessions were held during December, we discussed Kwanzaa (the first fruits of the harvest). Kwanzaa is based on seven fundamental principles called the Nguzo Saba (Karanga, 1977). These are Umoja (unity), Kujichagulia (self-determination), Ujima (collective work and responsibility), Ujamma (cooperative economics), Nia (purpose), Kuumbia (creativity), and Imani (faith).

While our sessions focused on African American culture, it may also be helpful to discuss aspects of disability culture, depending upon the group. Participants can explore values and assumptions they hold with other members of their disability group and how these values impact their attitudes and behaviors.

Session Seven: Final Session (What Have I Gained from This Program?)

The final session is a review session. In this session members can reflect upon what the program has meant to them. Generally, by the seventh session, the group has become a supportive resource for group members, and the group is functioning as a cohesive unit. Members will typically show concern and positive regard for members individually and collectively. If evaluation data are collected, it should be at the end of this session.

SUMMARY

This chapter provided general guidelines for running a social support group. Group objectives must be well defined and clear. Recruitment and retention efforts must be attended to. The structure of the sessions must be developed so as to facilitate the group's meeting its goal. The program content must be relevant and of value to participants. Critical to the success of the intervention is that consumers with disabilities be involved in substantial ways. The social support groups this author has run have been enjoyable and beneficial to consumers and staff alike. Group members met their objective of learning how to access and use social support. In doing so, improvements in mental health and vocational outcomes were realized.

8

Empowering African Americans Through Increasing Perceptions of Control and Self-efficacy Beliefs

In chapter 6, a rationale for the importance of psychological control and self-efficacy beliefs for enhancing outcomes for African Americans with chronic illnesses and disabilities was provided. As discussed in that chapter, perceptions of psychological control and self-efficacy beliefs are intrapersonal resources that can help one to achieve desired goals and to function adaptively. These intrapersonal resources are empowering for everyone and especially for individuals who may not have material or tangible resources. In this chapter, I outline strategies that can be used to increase self-efficacy beliefs and perceptions of psychological control among African Americans with chronic illnesses and disabilities. The strategies outlined in this chapter can be utilized by consumers and/or by professionals who work with consumers.

Psychological control and self-efficacy are expected to lead to more positive outcomes and a higher level of adaptive functioning. Many of these strategies have been used in interventions with African Americans with disabilities and chronic illnesses.

OVERVIEW OF EMPOWERMENT INTERVENTION

As noted in chapter 7, working with colleagues, I have developed, implemented, and evaluated several intervention programs aimed at improving or enhancing mental health, functional, and vocational outcomes for African Americans with disabilities. In this chapter, I discuss strategies used in a most recent intervention that was targeted at changing self-efficacy beliefs and perceptions of control in order to improve mental health (i.e., decrease depression) and vocational outcomes (e.g., become gainfully employed) among a group of working-age African Americans with disabilities.

The intervention was designed to achieve the following objectives: (1) to increase positive perceptions of self, (2) to increase goal-setting behavior, (3) to increase the perception of control in one's life and to learn to distinguish between what one can and cannot control, (4) to improve participants' self-efficacy beliefs, and (5) to increase the recognition and utilization of adaptive coping strategies for achieving desired outcomes. The objectives and tasks used to meet the objectives were interrelated in that improvements in one area were expected to relate to improvements in other areas. For example, goal setting should increase one's self-efficacy beliefs and utilization of adaptive coping strategies. African Americans who participated in the intervention had varied disabilities, including physical, chronic illness, substance abuse, and cognitive disabilities (among others).

The procedures for bringing group members together and beginning the intervention sessions were similar to those used for initiating the social support group discussed in the previous chapter. The reader is referred to chapter 7 for a discussion of strategies for recruiting and retaining group participants, and selecting facilitators.

There were twelve participants and two facilitators in this group. All participants were African American and had a disability. Both facilitators were African American, and one of the facilitators had a physical disability. Group members differed in some personal characteristics; however, the intervention was based on the assumption that there were some perceived similarity and common interests and values. To this end, although group members differed in type of disability, gender, and age, there were several similarities. They were all consumers of Rehabilitation Services Administration. They were all unemployed and seeking work and all were within a working-age range (i.e., less than 55). They were all African American and all lived in the same section of the city. Importantly they all came together with a common goal of finding employment.

The intervention was facilitated via a group structure deemed important for facilitating group process and outcomes. Within a group, members can provide feedback and support to one another and help each other to achieve individual and group goals. As with the social support intervention, sessions were conducted in a culturally congruent manner.

The group met consequently for seven sessions for about 2.5 hours once a week. During the first two sessions, members developed rules and norms for how the group would function. For example, one norm was to recognize the accomplishment of each person over the previous week. Other sessions were devoted more specifically to the achievement of the project's objectives (i.e., skill development through directed and supportive activities and exercises).

Initial Strategies for Strengthening Feelings of Control

An important first step in developing self-efficacy and psychological control is to acquaint individuals with the idea that they have some control in their lives. The concept of control may be elusive for people who have been historically disenfranchised and oppressed (a characterization of many members of our group). Members of this group were of low socioeconomic status, without money and jobs, and with limited access to material resources. However, this did not mean that these individuals were without control. As will be discussed, control is dependent upon one's conceptualization of what it means to have and not have it.

We introduced the notion of control by having group members think about how their past actions have affected their outcomes. We used a "victim" versus "doer" paradigm to facilitate an understanding of the person's perception of his or her role in being a victim or a doer. The objective of the discussion was to get people to begin to see that they have a choice in whether they see themselves as a victim or a doer. One's perceptions or views of herself as a victim or doer will directly affect choices that are made.

In one exercise, we had people generate a list of positive and negative events that had happened over the past month and then provide an explanation for the cause of these events. These lists were shared among group members. By examining their lists, individuals could begin to examine the reasons for their outcomes. They could begin to see a pattern in their behavior and the role of their behavior in outcomes across diverse situations. For example, one person recounted the negative outcome of not having anyone to celebrate her birthday with and another negative outcome of not having anyone to baby-sit while she went to an appointment. There are several potential reasons for these outcomes. In examining the reason for not having anyone to celebrate her birthday with, significant others may have been busy, no one may have known it was her birthday, or perhaps no one wanted to be with this person on her birthday. In trying to understand why this occurred, the individual and group members began to see how the explanation for this particular outcome is similar to the explanation for other outcomes. Then they began to see convergence within the person's behavior and how this behavior produces similar outcomes across diverse situations. In this case, perhaps, there was something about the person's actions that contributed to her negative outcomes in both situations. For example, maybe this individual did not inform people that it was her birthday early on or that she needed a sitter. Or perhaps she expected people to volunteer, when in fact she may have needed to ask. We observed that if the individual could not personally see the pattern or connection between her behavior and outcomes, group members could and were certain to point them out.

To take another example, we asked people in our group to examine the causes of their unemployment. One individual believed that she was unemployed because employers discriminate against people with disabilities. She felt that since she had no power to control who discriminates, there was little she could do in terms of securing employment. While discrimination against people with disabilities unfortunately does exist, this thinking may lead to a victim mentality—i.e., someone "discriminates against me—thereby doing something to me that I have no control over." Another individual reported that she believed she was unemployed because she didn't have marketable skills. Both discrimination and lack of marketable skills are plausible reasons for being unemployed. However, the person who reported discrimination as the reason is more likely to feel like a victim than the person who reported that she didn't have marketable skills because it is more difficult to change others' behavior than the behavior of self. What could these individuals do? The first person could inform discriminating employers that discrimination against people with disabilities is illegal and take possible legal action (i.e., file a discrimination suit). The second person could gain marketable skills. In both cases these individuals become doers. For both situations, we emphasized that whatever their situation, something can be done about it. In both situations we also emphasized making realistic and practical choices. For example, filing a discrimination suit may not be practical or realistic for a person who felt she was being discriminated against, but one simple action might be to ask for and review a copy of the personnel policy, including the anti-discrimination policy. If an individual felt she could not gain employment because she did not have marketable skills, one task might be to figure out what skills she did have that are marketable.

When people feel that they have little choice in what happens because of discrimination, life circumstances, health, and medical conditions, they will not put in effort to change their condition. In fact, it would be counterintuitive to try to change a situation if one believed that she did not have any influence or power in effecting change.

This is not to say that all members of this group were powerless and without perceived control. Quite the opposite. Members of this group were African American, unemployed, with very little money or material resources. Many had experienced situations in which, because of life circumstances, they were not in control of day-to-day or long-term outcomes. But we found that many of these individuals were doers and not victims in general. In spite of what could be considered oppressive life circumstances, they had not given up or subjugated control totally to others, to luck, or fate. These individuals had learned to use adaptive and empowering thought patterns. Our intention in the group was to augment and support these patterns, to develop these patterns in members who had not acquired them, and to have the adaptive thinker's model and show the maladaptive thinkers how it could be done.

Therefore, in our group we spent a great deal of time discussing what it means not to be a victim. To be a victim subjugates control outside of the self. To be a doer liberates oneself. We discussed the fact that there may be little choice in whether a life situation exists (i.e., loss of job, traumatic injury, chronicity of disease, being born poor, etc.), but we have a choice in how we react to the condition or situation. We have a choice in how we feel and what we think about a given situation. In our groups, members shared their own efforts to be doers rather than victims under aversive conditions. Consistent with Africentric worldview, they shared how they had learned to turn a negative into a positive and to make a way out of no way.

Closely related to the victim and doer dichotomy is the concept of internal and external locus of control. Discussions in our group centered around helping members to understand the concepts of internality and externality and what these mean in the person's life. As discussed in chapter 6, *internality* refers to the belief in one's ability to control reinforcement for one's actions, outcomes, and consequences. It refers to how much responsibility one assumes for what happens in one's life (internal) as opposed to believing that others or external circumstances determine what happens in one's life (*externality*). The essential question of internality versus externality is whether or not I believe positive or negative reinforcements are derived from my actions or outside of my control. For example, a person with an internal orientation may believe that if she applies to enough jobs (behavior), she will eventually find employment (positive reinforcement or reward) and if she doesn't apply for jobs, she will not obtain employment (negative reinforcement). A person with an external orientation may believe that even if she applies for several jobs (behavior), obtaining employment will mostly be a matter of fate or luck (external).

A history of discrimination and oppression in this country have created circumstances under which African Americans may not have been rewarded even when they put in hard work and effort. For example, the individual may not have been rewarded with a job even after several job applications have been submitted. Or a person may not have been able to attend college even after studying hard and getting good grades in high school. Or a person may have not been able to move into a good neighborhood even after obtaining a good education and employment. It is not difficult to see how external beliefs about reinforcement may develop within African Americans. Externality develops from contexts in which there have been prior experiences of inconsistent reinforcement (either rewards and punishment). Often these internal and external beliefs are developed from childhood and become a trait, or part of the individual's personality. In order for African Americans to learn to resist an external orientation, a discussion of why these beliefs exist may be necessary. In our group, all members could provide examples of how effort and ability had not paid off. However, they could also provide examples of where it had.

Internality leads one to adopt a doer mentality, and externality leads one to adopt a victim mentality. In cases where individuals may be disadvantaged with no job, money, or material resources, it may be natural to feel like a victim and forget that one can take an active role in determining life's outcomes. Discussing these concepts and practicing these skills with other group members is helpful. Within an environment where there are similar others who can provide information about their own efforts to be active and take control, transformation from being a victim to being a doer can occur. The experience of other group members normalizes aversive and oppressive experiences and reinforces to the individual that some types of control is possible.

Victim mentality and external beliefs promote defeatism and helplessness. Therefore, emphasizing the things that one can do is essential. In our groups we emphasized that we might not always have a choice over all aspects of our life, (i.e., whether or not we are a wheelchair user, what ethnic or racial group we belong to), but we do have a choice regarding other important aspects, (i.e., where we choose to go, whom we choose to interact with, how we choose to feel about ourselves, and what types of thoughts we choose to have). Only the individual can choose whether or not she or he feels like a victim or a doer. No one else can control one's own feelings and thoughts.

Of note is that the discussion of these concepts is likely to be more effective when done within a group of similar others rather than in a one-on-one setting such as might occur with a professional. Group members provide the framework for giving support and encouraging adaptive beliefs. Group members can share their experiences of both failure and success and serve as models for each other. Group members help in the interpretation and analysis of behaviors and consequences. Finally, other group members provide affirmation and positive regard.

In our group, we explained how feelings of being in and out of control, victims or doers, or internal versus external affect goal attainment. The point was made that goals cannot be attained when one is a victim and when one has an external orientation. Victims have no control and therefore cannot effect change. Goal attainment is virtually impossible when one is a victim. Doers, on the other hand, will continue to be active and make some choices even under adverse circumstances.

The link between one's feeling of being a doer/internal versus victim/external is especially important for persons to make if they are in situations where their desired outcomes are long-term, challenging, and difficult to achieve. A good example is in the employment arena. Months of searching for a job and remaining unemployed may lead the individual to feel like a victim and then to subsequently think and act like a victim. Here continued unemployment exacerbates negative emotions (e.g., anxiety, fear), which contributes to maladaptive thoughts ("I have been looking for so long, I will never get a job") which leads to poor job-search strategies (behaviors). This is a vicious cycle, with poor job-search strategies contributing to negative emotional states and so on. However, in the mind of the doer, the person can tell herself, "I didn't get the job, but at least I tried, and the job-search experience has taught me an additional skill to use" (i.e., how to seek out jobs). After evaluating one's personal efforts and affective and cognitive reactions, the person can also begin to identify external obstacles to securing employment (i.e., job market, transportation, etc.).

The link between being a doer and goal attainment can also be used to discuss examples of racism and discrimination against persons with disabilities and discrimination against African Americans. For example, our group discussed the fact that I may not be able to control who discriminates against me, but I can control how I react to it and what I do about it.

Learning to set goals is critical in the empowerment process. It is essential to feeling in control and being responsible for one's actions. Goal setting leads us to behave in ways that will facilitate desired outcomes. Goal setting is but one of several steps for developing self-efficacious beliefs as suggested by self-efficacy theory (Bandura 1986; Maddux, 1996). Goal setting will be discussed followed by a discussion of other strategies that can be used to increase self-efficacy, including guided mastery experiences, modeling, relaxation, and persuasion. These steps have been nicely described by Maddux and Lewis (1995) and applications to people with disabilities and chronic illnesses are made here.

DEVELOPING SELF-EFFICACY BELIEFS

Goal Setting

Goal setting is an essential first step in the movement toward empowerment. Although goal setting seems intuitive and simple, it is not a trivial exercise. Many individuals have learned to function in a goalless and reactive manner rather than a goal-directed and proactive manner. Previous history and experience have reinforced the mind-set of not setting goals when they most likely will not be met.

The absence of goal-setting behavior may especially be the case with individuals who have been oppressed, disadvantaged, and/or discriminated against. These individuals may have learned that goal setting may not always be productive and in fact may be a waste of time. Under circumstances of oppression and discrimination, things happen to a person rather than the person controlling what happens or making something happen.

However, goal setting can be learned, even among individuals who have not lived in a culture where goal setting is a cultural norm. An important first step in goal setting is to learn how to set realistic goals. Realistic goals are attainable, practical, concrete, and individualized. Goals should also be time defined. The goal of obtaining a graduate degree may not be attainable within the time desired by a given person, but having the goal to enroll in a specific training course may be. Goals should not be so difficult that attaining them are impossible nor so easy that little effort has to be put into reaching them. Goals should also be individualized. In our group, each member identified a goal they wanted to reach after six months. These goals were used as a starting point for discussing the practicality and attainability of goals.

Once a goal has been specified, smaller subgoals should be delineated. The goal of many members in our group was to obtain employment. Therefore, several smaller goals had to be realized before the employment goal could be met. For example, a subgoal might be as simple as scheduling rehabilitation and medical appointments at the appropriate time period. A second subgoal might be to learn how to use public transportation to get to these appointments. A more complex long-term goal might be to find suitable employment. Each of these small goals will need to be met before the larger one can be achieved.

We can also set cognitive and affective goals, along with behavioral or action-oriented goals. For example, an affective goal may be to decrease one's negative thinking pattern following an aversive situation. If I don't get a job, I will be able to control my anxiety (affective goal) and not view myself as worthless (cognitive goal). As with behavioral self-efficacy, strategies can be used to increase cognitive and affective self-efficacy by identifying cognitive and affective goals (Maddux & Lewis, 1995). Cognitive and affective subgoals, along with behavioral subgoals, can be used to reach larger goals. For example, one affective subgoal may be to repeat an affirmation to oneself each day. Another may be to think about a pleasant experience whenever one starts to feel anxious.

A suggestion is to write down one's goals and subgoals. The process of writing down goals makes them more real in the person's mind. Reviewing and referring to these goals every day is also helpful. Sharing written goals with significant others should also reinforce and provide support for reaching goals.

Following the identification of a goal, the next step is to develop a plan to carry out these goals. Through extensive practice one begins to act on that goal. Guided mastery experiences (practice) can be used to achieve desired outcomes and is discussed next.

Guided Mastery Experiences

One way to strengthen self-efficacy is through guided mastery experiences. This involves breaking a task into small, incremental steps that can be done within a relatively short period of time (Bandura, 1986). These tasks should be directed at achieving subgoals. For example subtasks related to meeting employment subgoals were described previously (i.e., schedule appointment, read help-wanted ads, learn to use public transportation, etc.). Once a subtask is accomplished, another is added until the desired behavior is achieved and the overall goal has been met.

For example, if the overall goal is to find suitable housing, one first step might be to learn how to read a housing ad. A second step might be to learn how to complete a housing application. The third step might be to learn how to carry out an interview with the landlord. It may not be the most effective strategy to set the goal of finding suitable housing as the first goal because failure and disappointment may erode one's confidence, which is likely to erode self-efficacy beliefs. On the contrary, small tasks that are successfully completed contribute to one's feelings of accomplishment and promote self-efficacy beliefs. Such feelings are likely to lead to more positive emotional and affective states and more confidence that one can successfully accomplish a task.

When tasks are selected, they should be progressive in level of difficulty. Initial tasks should not be so difficult that they guarantee failure nor so easy that accomplishment is meaningless. For example, if the person has already had extensive experience completing housing applications, this subgoal may not be challenging enough. The level of difficulty set for the task should depend upon the individual's prior experiences with goal setting and with accomplishing goals. Under conditions where the individual has extensive goal-setting experience and has successfully completed desired goals, initial task difficulty should be harder than when experience is limited.

Support from others will also help in goal attainment. The beneficial nature of support and strategies for increasing support were discussed in the previous chapter and will be returned to later in this chapter. Supportive others can provide information to assist in the completion of tasks (i.e., where there is a job opening). Supportive others can provide material resources (i.e., transportation to an interview appointment or child-care assistance). Finally, supportive others can provide affirmation of one's worth and competence especially during stressful times. Such affirmation is critical to continuing goal-directive behaviors, especially following periods of failure.

Modeling

One does not always have to be personally involved in practice and guided mastery of tasks to develop self-efficacy. Modeling is another mechanism for increasing self-efficacy. Social modeling involves observing others engaged in the desired behaviors. When seeking employment, we can observe and learn from others how to read an employment ad, how to use public transportation, and how to act on an interview.

When models are used in training sessions, they are most effective when the model is as similar to the participant as possible. Similarity between the model and the observer makes the accomplishment of desired goal seem possible—"if this person can do it, so can I." For persons with a disability and/or chronic illness, a model with a similar disability and chronic illness would be more effective than one without.

Another consideration for African Americans is that the model be someone with similar values and worldview. As discussed in chapter 3, cultural values such as interdependence, communalism, and spirituality are important to many African Americans and may be useful as criteria for selecting models. In this setting, perceived similarity and the relationship one has with the model may be as important a consideration as technical expertise. Here, for example, having a model demonstrate what she did to seek employment may be more effective than having an employment counselor provide job-seeking tips. All things being equal, an effective model for an African American person with a disability would be another African American with the same type of disability and values.

Guided Imagery

Guided imagery may also be used to increase self-efficacy beliefs and subsequently facilitate desired outcomes. Individuals can learn how to visualize themselves as behaving in desired ways. In our group, we had individuals imagine how they would feel, think, and act if they were employed.

Guided imagery can also be used to help persons through an aversive or negative situation. If the interview process is perceived as stressful, individuals can learn to go through the procedure in their minds in gradual steps (i.e., leave home, catch a bus to the site, enter the building, talk to the receptionist, etc.). Guided imagery may be facilitated by having a leader introduce successive steps to the person, who follows along in her mind.

Relaxation, meditation, and other stress-reducing techniques can be done in connection with guided imagery and other mastery techniques. When individuals are relaxed and calm, they are able to think more clearly, and effectively, and to make better decisions.

Persuasion

Oftentimes, people engage in desired behaviors because they are persuaded to or told to by someone who has influence over them. This influence can be based on respect, liking, or power from the other person. Thus *persuasion* is another mechanism for increasing self-efficacy. Persuasion occurs when one person influences another to think or behave in a certain manner. Persuasion can be accomplished by providing knowledge and information in areas where knowledge and information may be needed to accomplish a goal. For example, telling the individual where there are job openings and requesting that they go and check them out is persuasion. As with modeling, persuasion will be more effective if there is similarity between the persuader and the person who is persuaded. Persuasion, like modeling, is also more effective when mutual respect and liking between the persuader and the persuaded exist. When a person changes his behavior because he likes and respects the persuader, behavioral change is likely to be internalized and not disappear when the persuader is no longer around.

Persuasion must be done in a manner that is accessible and congruent with the target person's values, norms, and language. For African Americans, a formal or highly structured presentation by a persuader on how to conduct a job interview may by less effective than experiential sessions in which the individual talks more informally about the experience of going on a job interview.

As with modeling, the credibility of the persuader is contingent upon the person's ability to relate to and connect at an interpersonal level. The absence of an interpersonal relationship may account for some of the lack of persuasion or nonadherence of African Americans to recommended medical or rehabilitation services and treatment by Whites. A technical or expert basis for persuasion may not be effective in the absence of such an interpersonal relationship. Thus, as a consumer, I may not necessarily comply to prescribed appointments because you tell me to based on your status as the expert, but because I like and respect you, and I want to do what you think is right. Characteristics of the persuader then are a consideration in selecting professionals who provide services and health care to consumers with disabilities and chronic illnesses. Our group had an individual with a physical disability function as a persuader. This individual was perceived as very credible, and group members were persuaded because they liked and respected her.

Social Support

Another strategy for increasing self-efficacy and adaptive coping is through the provision of social support. Social support for desired change is important and must come not only from within a specific behavioral change environment (such as from an employment counselor), but throughout the individual's socioenvironmental context (i.e., at home, church, and within other circles). The support of family and friends is important in this regard.

The utilization of social support within an informal environment is culturally congruent for African Americans, who may value communal and interpersonal relationships. Self-efficacy interventions that build upon these natural relationships are expected to be more effective than those that do not. Strategies for increasing social support were considered in chapter 7.

When Desired Goals Cannot Be Met

Much of the discussion of the development of self-efficacy beliefs has centered on the mastery of tasks involving practice in order to increase feelings and judgments of accomplishments toward the attainment of desired goals. What can be done when one cannot realistically expect to achieve a desired goal because of personal or environmental circumstances (i.e., a disability that is very severe or the lack of material resources)? Under these circumstances, other types of control must be considered.

In this case, emotion-focused control may be used to change one's thoughts and beliefs surrounding a particular situation. For example, a person with a severe disability may not be able to work outside the home. However, this person can change the meaning of work for him or her so that the absence of work is not perceived negatively. Exercises and activities can be devoted to examine other important values (i.e., family, spirituality, love, etc.).

Acceptance

Acceptance can be a powerful strategy for psychological control. Acceptance does not necessarily mean that the person has been defeated or has given up, but that the person can accept what he or she cannot change and move on to focus on what can be changed. When this happens, the person is no longer putting his efforts into something that will not help him to accomplish desired goals. In our group we found it necessary to review priorities and values so that individuals could see what was and was not important and how their values could be reflected given their current situation.

Discussions of acceptance may be especially important for individuals who have been stigmatized on the basis of disability or ethnicity. When we look to the larger world for information about how we should look and act, we are less likely to be accepting of our personal circumstances. Acceptance and the serenity that goes with it have to be achieved at an individual level. Acceptance may be derived from one's faith and spiritual beliefs.

Spirituality

Spiritual beliefs may be adaptive and are discussed in this chapter because of the centrality of spirituality to African Americans. People of African descent are spiritual people. Spiritual beliefs provide a type of secondary control in that control is not to fate or luck, but to a higher power. As discussed in chapter 3, research has shown spiritual beliefs to aid in effective coping for African Americans. African Americans with higher levels of spirituality have better outcomes than those with lower levels of spirituality. Spiritual rituals such as attending church or mosque, reading the Koran or Bible, praying, and meditation may help one accept life circumstances and grow stronger under aversive conditions.

Spirituality may be especially conducive when there is no plausible explanation for an adverse outcome. Faith in a greater power provides a framework for dealing with the unexplainable. Knowing that there is a force greater than self that shapes our destiny is empowering. In our group sessions, we encouraged the expression of spirituality. In one group, each session began with a prayer, and members offered prayers for the success of each other. Expression of spirituality in whatever form it takes should be encouraged and supported.

The use of spirituality as a coping strategy may run counter to those approaches that are more behaviorally oriented and scientifically based. Therefore, group facilitators and professionals may need training in being sensitive to the importance of spirituality for African Americans.

SUMMARY

Perceptions of psychological control and self-efficacy beliefs can be powerful intrapersonal resources for behavioral change. Having a victim/external orientation is not conducive to goal setting and achievement. Goal setting, the first step in developing self-efficacy is important and attainable goals should be set. Goals are more likely to be reached by specifying subgoals. Once goals have been set, there are several strategies that can be used to increase efficacy, including guided mastery or practice. With guided mastery, the individual engages in incremental steps. The accomplishments of each small step reinforce feelings and thoughts of mastery and competency. Modeling, persuasion, and guided imagery can also be used to increase self-efficacy beliefs. These can be augmented by using stress-reducing techniques such as relaxation and exercise. When there are situations where there is no realistic chance of change, then modifying one's thoughts and feelings is a way of gaining control. Here reinterpretation of the situation and acceptance are adaptive. Spiritual beliefs also provide a framework for acceptance when negative outcomes occur.

The ability to actively plan, to set and carry out realistic goals, to develop self-efficacious beliefs and to learn to accept what one cannot control can empower African Americans with disabilities and chronic illnesses.

9

Conclusions and Directions for Future Work

This book was written to fill a need for more relevant information on African Americans with chronic illnesses and disabilities. Despite the high prevalence of disability in the African American community, relatively little has been written. One purpose in writing this book was simply to increase awareness about disability and chronic illness and the status of African Americans with disabilities and chronic illness. The aim was to make salient how disability and chronic illness affect most African Americans in this country. A second purpose was to provide an examination of research (albeit limited) on factors that promote both adaptive and maladaptive functioning and adjustment. As discussed throughout this book, poor adjustment and outcomes are not inevitable, and many African Americans with disabilities and chronic illnesses function quite well. Certain psychological, social, environmental, and cultural factors contribute to adjustment and have been explicated throughout the book.

A third purpose was to discuss the influence of culture in the African American disability and chronic illness experience. Limited research has addressed the unique culture of African Americans, and even less discusses the impact of culture on the experience of disability and chronic illness. Africentric values provide the framework for discussing the culture of African Americans in this book.

Finally, but perhaps most importantly, the book attempts to provide examples of successful programs and strategies that African Americans with disabilities and chronic illnesses can use. The programs and strategies discussed were based on the work of the author and colleagues, but they seem promising for others' use, including consumer groups and disability and rehabilitation organizations.

A central theme throughout the book is that programs and strategies must be culturally congruent. This involves using the values, norms, and beliefs of African Americans, involving consumers with disabilities, and having an appropriate theoretical framework when conducting research and developing programs.

As with other efforts that arise out of a scarcity of information on an important topic, this book raises several questions and points to areas of needed research and program development. The comments, thoughts, and suggestions that follow are offered as challenges to others who are committed to understanding and improving the quality of life and the conditions of African Americans with chronic illnesses and disabilities.

SUGGESTIONS FOR FUTURE EFFORTS

Chapter 1 highlighted disparities in morbidity, mortality, disability, and chronic illness by comparing African Americans to Whites. African Americans are less likely to engage in preventive health practices, receive routine medical care, and participate in rehabilitation services and programs than Whites. Differences remain even when socioeconomic factors are controlled for. Differential patterns of health, medical, and rehabilitation utilization account for many of these disparities. Psychological, social, and cultural factors also contribute to these differences.

However, we need to know much more about the demography and status of disability and chronic illness among African Americans. We know, for example, that the average individual who is disabled is likely to be female, single, of low socioeconomic status, and unemployed (Walker, Saravanabhavan, Williams, Brown, & West, 1996). We also know, for example, that African Americans who reside in the inner city have additional stressors that contribute to mortality and morbidity. We need to find out more about other African American groups who are at higher risk for mortality and morbidity. Who are these individuals, and what risk factors contribute to their higher mortality and morbidity? Research on environmental factors that lead to increased morbidity and disability is needed, along with research on interpersonal or psychological factors.

For example, a disability we need to know more about is traumatic spinal cord injury. There has been an increase in the prevalence of traumatic spinal cord injury among young African American males over the past decade. The growing number of severe traumatic spinal cord injuries occur among young African American males who reside in the inner cities. These injuries are for the most part due to gunshot wounds. Involvement in drug behaviors and a risky lifestyle are implicated in many of these traumatic injuries, although in some situations innocent bystanders who happened to be in the wrong place at the wrong time are injured. These males are quite young at the time of injury—often under the age of 21, with many years ahead of them. More systematic study of this population is needed. What psychological and environmental factors contribute to the higher incidence of traumatic injuries among African American males who reside in inner cities? What can be done to decrease these injuries? What can be done to promote adaptive functioning among these individuals?

Another example of a subject needing additional research and program is in the area of AIDS infection. The incidence of AIDS cases continues to increase in the African American community even as there is leveling off of new AIDS cases among some populations (e.g., gay White males). The growth is seen especially among young African American females. What risk factors contribute to the spread of HIV infection among African American females, and what are the age groups at which infection are most likely to occur? How can we assist African Americans living with AIDS to function optimally?

These are but two examples of chronic illnesses and disabilities where more research and programmatic efforts are needed. There are, of course, many others. These conditions were selected because they have profound costs to the individual, family, community, and society. The costs of these conditions are disproportionally borne by the African American community. Both of these conditions affect relatively young populations who, with appropriate environmental resources and supports can be productive. More research is needed on how to prevent these and other preventable conditions and how to improve the quality of life for individuals with these conditions.

In an attempt to be broad and inclusive, this book has viewed disability very generally, but study on specific disability groups is clearly warranted and encouraged. As the two cited disabling conditions illustrate, functioning and adjustment are expected to differ for different disability groups based on factors such as the chronicity of the condition, the functional limitations imposed by the condition, and even the stigma (i.e., AIDS versus stroke) of the condition. Factors that affect the level of functioning or predictors are also expected to differ for different populations. Outcomes of interest would also differ depending upon the disability or chronic illness group. For example, among persons living with AIDS, certain drug therapies along with stress-reduction techniques are likely to be predictors of good functioning (e.g., T-cell counts). For individuals recovering from a traumatic spinal cord injury, physical therapy and role adjustment might be important to consider as predictors of functional ability (e.g., mobility). Understanding the specificity of a particular disability's predictors and outcomes is necessary in order to develop appropriate programs.

Mental illness and addiction as a disability and chronic condition were not extensively addressed in this book although individuals with mental illness and addiction constitute a substantial percentage of the population of individuals with disabilities. We need further discussion of mental illness and addiction and the consequences of such conditions among African Americans. More on the contributions of these conditions to physical disabilities and the concurrence of these conditions with other chronic conditions is also needed. For example, we know that drug addiction is associated with increased trauma, disability, and chronic conditions. We need more research devoted to understanding the interactions of these variables.

This book focused on the role of cultural factors in the experience of disability and chronic illness, maintaining that culture affects both whether or not disabilities and chronic illnesses are acquired and how well one adjusts to disability and chronic illness. The argument was made that Africentric values are adaptive in helping African Americans cope with disability and chronic illness. However, relatively little empirical work has been done on Africentric values among the general African American population. More research on Africentric values using diverse African American populations, that is, those with chronic illnesses and disabilities and those without, is needed. Much of the work that has been done on Africentric values has been limited to college students because they comprise a convenient population to study.

We also need to more clearly specify which components of an Africentric worldview are adaptive for African Americans with chronic illnesses and disabilities and which are not. For example, a communalism orientation may be helpful insofar as it fosters interdependence and support from others. However, communalism also dictates that one be a provider as well as a recipient of support. When an individual has to deal with stressors that may accompany his or her own adaptation to a disability, assuming responsibility for other members of the family or extended kin can bring on unwanted additional stress.

An understanding of the role of Africentric worldview in other disability and rehabilitation-related domains (e.g., acceptance of disability, adjustment to disability, quality of life) as well as domains outside rehabilitation (e.g., job success, parenting success) is also needed. Do individuals with Africentric values report a better quality of life than those without? Do individuals with Africentric values have greater acceptance of the disability? This research has implications for developing programs aimed at acknowledging or increasing Africentric values.

In this book, I discuss my research, which has focused on understanding the role of certain social and psychological factors in the functioning of African Americans with disabilities. Chapter 4 examines factors that contribute to successful employment, and chapter 5 examines the role of social support on mental health and vocational outcomes. The findings identify environmental (e.g., social support from others), psychological (e.g., positive self-perception), and demographic (e.g., prior work history, transportation) factors that contribute to positive or negative outcomes. While this research contributes to a better understanding of functioning, it is limited and does not fully elucidate all possible variables that might contribute to successful adjustment.

The identification of mental health and employment as indicators of functional outcomes is also limited as outcome variables, and other outcomes are worthy of examination. We need to know more about factors that impact success in other domains such as academic performance and school transition for younger populations of African Americans. As noted in chapter 1 and earlier in this chapter, the level of education is substantially lower for African Americans with disabilities than those without disabilities. Lower levels of education contribute negatively to employment opportunities, income potential, housing opportunity, and so on. What factors contribute to successful school achievement among young African Americans? What kinds of school to workplace initiatives would facilitate vocational adjustment among youth? What programs would be most effective in helping young consumers make a successful transition from school to work?

Disability and chronic illness affect nearly everyone, but most immediately one's family unit. We need to know more about the impact of having a chronic illness or disability on family members. Research on the African American family with a family member with a disability is needed given that African American families differ from the families of other ethnic groups. For example, a disability may strengthen a family unit by bringing family members together. On the other hand, a disability or a chronic illness can create additional stressors that are disruptive to the family. What are the conditions under which a disability increases resiliency, and what are the conditions under which it contributes to dysfunctional behavior?

In the research discussed in chapters 4 and 5, several significant statistical findings are reported. However, this research has some limitations based on methods used, and there is a need to improve the validity of this type of research. Data were obtained from consumer self-report, and the study designs were cross-sectional. Longitudinal and prospective studies that track the temporal sequencing of factors contributing to certain outcomes (i.e., employment, mental health) are necessary. That is, we need a clearer elucidation of the process of adjusting. This kind of methodology will be helpful when developing interventions for consumers. For example, at what point or during what time periods would programs be most helpful in the adjustment process? We also need models that can identify with good confidence who is and is not most likely to achieve favorable outcomes given cost considerations. We also need to know which programs work well for which groups.

More qualitative research, including interviews and case studies, are indicated. Interviews with successful African Americans with disabilities and chronic illnesses will be quite helpful in identifying factors that facilitated their successes. How were these individuals able to obtain their desired goals and accomplish what they wanted? This research would focus on resiliency among Africans with disabilities, not just pathology.

Two chapters (7 and 8) are devoted to discussing programs and strategies I have used with African American consumers to improve mental health and employment. These chapters are limited by my perspective. Much more research is needed on other successful programs with African American consumers. There has been very little in the rehabilitation literature on effective programs for African Americans with disabilities and chronic illnesses. Continued work evaluating the effectiveness of different intervention strategies and approaches is needed. For example, while I attempted to make a convincing (I hope) argument for the use of self-efficacious beliefs and other control beliefs, perhaps there are other strategies that would be equally or more effective with African Americans. This would involve identifying other theoretical frameworks around which to organize programs and strategies. It would also be of interest to investigate whether or not programs that use Africentric-based strategies (e.g., spirituality, communalism, interdependence) are more effective than those that do not.

Finally, we also need more consumer-led research. Consumers are in a position to offer a unique perspective. We need consumers to posit the questions that should be asked, the issues to be addressed, and the problems to be solved. In my work, I have focused on trying to understand and improve employment and mental health as indicators of levels of functioning. However, other questions may be equally important from the perspective of consumers. For example, what is needed to improve access to appropriate housing? What are the best ways or what methods should be used to address these questions?

While participatory action research methods were used in my research, it has been limited insofar as consumers have assumed secondary, not primary, responsibilities. Participatory action research would involve African American consumers in all phases and levels in research and programs. More participatory action research is needed in order for change to come from within and not be forced by outsiders. In this regard, we need more resources devoted to training consumers to become researchers and program developers.

To this end, we can perhaps best assist African American consumers with disabilities and chronic illnesses by lending our technical expertise to consumer programs. African Americans with disabilities should be in positions to define their research and implement their programs. This is a challenge I hope consumers will take on.

Many of the questions and suggestions for future research outlined here are complex; they involve addressing broad societal issues (i.e., education for Americans with disabilities) and are not offered carelessly here. They are offered to stimulate thinking in the many areas where much more information, research, and program development are needed.

References

Affleck, G., Urrows, S., Tennen, H., & Higgins, P. (1992). Daily coping pain from rheumatoid arthritis: Patterns and correlations. *Pain, 51,* 221–229.

Akbar, N. (1979). African roots of Black personality. In W. D. Smith, K. Burlew, M. Moseley, & W. Whitney (Eds.), *Reflections on Black psychology*. Washington, DC: American University Press.

Allegrante, J. P., MacKenzie, C. R., & Robbins, L. (1991). Hip fracture in older persons: Does self-efficacy based on intervention have a role in rehabilitation? *Arthritis Care and Research, 4,* 39–47.

Alston, R. J., & Mngadi, S. (1992). The interaction between disability status and the African American experience: Implications for rehabilitation counseling. *Journal of Applied Rehabilitation Counseling, 23,* 12–15.

Anderson, B. L., Kiecolt-Glaser, J. K., & Glaser, R. (1994). A biobehavioral model of cancer stress and disease course. *American Psychologists, 49,* 389–404.

Anderson, L. (1991). Acculturative stress: A theory of relevance to Black Americans. *Clinical Psychology, 11,* 685–702.

Asante, M. K. (1988). *Afrocentricity*. Trenton, NJ: Africa World Press.

Asbury, C. A., Walker, S., Maholmes, V., Rackley, R., & White, S. (1991). *Prevalence and demographic association among race/ethnic minority populations in the United States: Implications for the 21st century*. Washington, DC: Howard University, Howard University Research and Training Center for Access to Rehabilitation and Economic Opportunity.

Atkins, B. (1988). An asset-oriented approach to cross-cultural issues: Blacks in rehabilitation. *Journal of Applied Rehabilitation Counseling, 19,* 45–49.

Azibo, D. A. (1989). African-centered theses on mental health and a nosology of Black/African personality disorder. *Journal of Black Psychology, 15,* 173–214.

Azibo, D. A. (1996). *African psychology in historical perspective: related commentary.* Trenton, NJ, African World Press.

Bailey, E. J. (1990). Health care use patterns among Detroit African Americans, 1910–1939. *Journal of the National Medical Association, 22,* 721–730.

Baldwin, J. A. (1990). African (black) psychology: Issues and synthesis. In R. L. Jones (Ed.), *Black psychology.* Berkeley, CA: Cobb & Henry.

Baldwin, J. A. (1981). Notes on an Africentric theory of Black personality testing. *Western Journal of Black Studies, 5,* 172–179.

Ball, R. E. (1983). Family and friends: A supportive network for low-income American Black families. *Journal of Comparative Family Studies, 14,* 51–65.

Bandura, A. (1990). Perceived self-efficacy in the exercise of control over AIDS infection. *Evaluation and Program Planning, 13,* 9–17.

Bandura, A. (1986). *Social foundations of thought and action: A social cognitive theory.* Englewood Cliffs, NJ: Prentice-Hall.

Bandura, A. (1977). *Social learning theory.* Englewood Cliffs, NJ: Prentice-Hall.

Barrera, M. (1986). Distinctions between social support concepts, measures, and models. *American Journal of Community Psychology, 14,* 413–445.

Barrera, M. (1981). Social support in the adjustment of pregnant adolescents. In B. H. Gottlieb (Ed.), *Social Networks and Social Support* (pp. 69–96). Beverly Hills: Sage.

Barrera, M., Sandler, I. M., & Ramsay, T. B. (1981). Preliminary development of a scale of social support: Studies on college students. *American Journal of Community Psychology, 9,* 435–447.

Beals, A. R. (1967). *Culture in process.* New York: Rinehart & Winston.

Beck, A. T., Steer, R. A., Garbin, M. C. (1988). Psychometric properties of the Beck Depression Inventory: Twenty-five years of evaluation. *Clinical Psychology, 8,* 77–100.

Belgrave, F. Z. (1991). Psychological predictors of adjustment to disability in African Americans. *Journal of Rehabilitation, 57,* 37–40.

Belgrave, F. Z., Davis, A., & Vadja, J. (1994). An examination of social support source, type, and satisfaction among African Americans and White Americans with disabilities. *Journal of Social Behavior and Personality, 9,* 307–320.

Belgrave, F. Z., & Lewis, D. M. (1994). The role of social support in compliance and other health behaviors for African Americans with chronic illnesses. *Journal of Health and Social Policy, 5,* 55–68.

Belgrave, F. Z., & Walker, S. (1991a). Differences in rehabilitation service utilization patterns of African Americans and White Americans with disabilities. In S. Walker, F. Z. Belgrave, R. Nicholls, and K. Turner (Eds.), *Future frontiers in the employment of minority persons with disabilities.* Washington, DC: Howard University Research and Training Center for Access to Rehabilitation and Economic Opportunity.

Belgrave, F. Z., & Walker, S. (1991b). Predictors of employment outcome of Black persons with disabilities. *Rehabilitation Psychology, 36,* 110–119.

Belgrave, F. Z., Walker, S., & Asbury, C. (1995). Variables related to vocational success among African Americans with disabilities. Unpublished manuscript. Available from Faye Z. Belgrave, Department of Psychology, Virginia Commonwealth University, Richmond, Virginia, 23284–2018.

Belgrave, F. Z., & Washington, A. (1986). Locus of control in chronically ill adolescents. *Journal of Rehabilitation, 51*, 53–57.

Bowe, F. (1985). Black adults with disabilities. A statistical report drawn from census bureau data. Washington, DC: Government Printing Office, 1984.

Bowe, F. (1991). *Black adults with disabilities: A portrait.* Report prepared for the President's Committee on Employment of People with Disabilities. Washington, DC: GPO.

Brown, D. R., & Gary, L. E. (1987). Stressful life events, social support networks, and physical and mental health of urban Black adults. *Journal of Human Stress, 13*, 165–174.

Brown, R. T., Doepke, K. J., & Kaslow, N. J. (1993). Risk-resistance adaptation model for pediatric chronic illness: Sickle cell syndrome as an example. *Clinical Psychology Review, 13*, 119–132.

Burlew, A. K., Belgrave, F. Z., Thorington, B., Barbarin, O., Telfair, J., & Kaluenia, J. (1995). Factors that influence psychosocial functioning in adults with sickle cell disease. Unpublished manuscript. Available from first author at the Department of Psychology, University of Cincinnati, Cincinnati, Ohio 45221.

Burns, R. (1997). Mammography's double standard. *Shape*, February 1997, p. 34.

Carver, C. S., Scheier, M., & Weintraub, J. K. (1989). Assessing coping strategies: A theoretical based approach. *Journal of Personality and Social Psychology, 56*, 267–283.

Cauce, A., Felner, R., & Primavera, J. (1982). Social support in high risk adolescents: structural components and adaptive impact. *American Journal of Community Psychology*, 10, 417–428.

Centers for Disease Control and Prevention. (1994). *Chronic Disease in Minority Populations.* U.S. Department of Health and Human Services, National Center for Chronic Disease Prevention and Health Promotion.

Chase, G. (1992). *African American students' use of family kin and non-kin supports and its impact on stress and adjustment.* Unpublished doctoral dissertation, George Washington University, Washington, DC.

Cheung, F. K., & Snowden, L. R. (1990). Community mental health and ethnic minority populations. *Community Mental Health Journal, 26*, 277–291.

Cicerone, K. D. (1991). Psychotherapy after mild traumatic brain injury: Relation to the nature and severity of subjective complaints. *Journal of Head Trauma Rehabilitation, 6*, 30–43.

Coates, D. L. (1985). Relationship between self-concept measures and social network characteristics of Black adolescents. *Journal of Early Adolescence, 5*, 319–338.

Cobb, J. (1976). Social support as a moderator of life stress. *Psychosomatic Medicine, 38*, 300–314.

Cohen, S. (1988). Psychosocial models of the role of social support in the etiology of physical disease. *Health Psychology, 7*, 269–297.

Cohen, S., & McKay G. (1984). Social support, stress and the buffering hypothesis: A theoretical analysis. In A. Baum, S. E. Taylor, & J. E. Singer (Eds.), *Handbook of Psychology and Health, Vol. IV* (pp. 253–267). Hilldale, NJ: Lawrence Erlbaum Associates.

Cohen, S., & Wills, T. A. (1985). Stress, social support, and the buffering hypothesis. *Psychological Bulletin, 98,* 310–357.

Covington, M. V., & Omelich, C. L. (1992). Self-efficacy and health behaviors. In R. Schwarzer (Ed.), *Self-efficacy: thought control of action.* Washington, DC: Hemisphere Publishing Corporation.

Crew, N. M., & Alhelstan, G. T. (1984). Functional assessment inventory manual. Menomonie: University of Wisconsin-Stout, Materials Development Center.

Devins, G. M., Binick, Y. M., Gorman, P., Dattell, M., McCloskey, B., Oscar, G., & Briggs, J. (1982). Perceived self-efficacy, outcome expectancies, and negative mood states in end-stage renal disease. *Journal of Abnormal Psychology, 91,* 241–244.

DiClemente, C., Fairhurst, S. K., & Piotrowski, N. A. (1996). Self-efficacy and addictive behaviors. In J. E. Maddux (Ed.), *Self-efficacy, adaptation, and adjustment.* New York: Plenum.

DiMatteo, M. R., & DiNicola, D. P. (1982). *Achieving patient compliance: The psychology of the medical practitioner's role.* New York: Pergamon.

Dolce, J. (1987). Self-efficacy and disability beliefs in behavioral treatment of pain. *Behavior Research and Therapy, 25,* 289–299.

Dressler, W. E. (1985). Extended family relationships, social support and mental health in a southern Black community. *Journal of Health and Social Behavior, 26,* 39–48.

Dressler, W. W., Dos-Santos, J. E., & Vileri, F. E. (1986). Blood pressure, ethnicity, and psychosocial resources. *Psychosomatic Medicine, 48,* 509–519.

Endo, R. (1984). Use of informal social networks for service-related information. *Psychological Reports, 54,* 354.

Esses, V. M., & Beaufoy, S. L. (1994). Determinants of attitudes toward people with disabilities. *Journal of Social Behavior and Personality, 9,* 43–64.

Ewart, C. K. (1992). Perceived self-efficacy in self-management of chronic disease. In R. Schwarzer (Ed.), *Self-efficacy: Thought control of action.* Washington, DC: Hemisphere Publishing Corporation.

Ewart, C. K. (1996). Self-efficacy and recovery from heart attack: Implications for a social-cognitive analysis of exercise and emotion. In J. E. Maddux (Ed.), *Self-efficacy, adaptation, and adjustment.* New York: Plenum.

Fisk, S. T., & Taylor, S. E. (1991). *Social cognition.* New York: McGraw-Hill.

Garland, H., Weinberg, R., Bruya, L., & Jackson, A. (1988). Self-efficacy and endurance performance: A longitudinal field test of cognitive mediation theory. *Applied Psychology: An International Review, 37,* 381–394.

Gattuso, S. M., Litt, M. D., & Fitzgerald, T. E. (1992). Coping with gastrointestinal endoscopy: Self-efficacy enhancement and coping styles. *Journal of Consulting Clinical Psychology, 60,* 133–139.

Gil, K. M. (1989). Coping with sickle cell disease pain. *Annals of Behavioral Medicine, 11,* 49–57.

Gil, K. M., Williams, D. A., Thompson, R. J., & Kinney, J. R. (1991). Sickle cell disease in children and adolescents: The relation of child and parent pain coping strategies on adjustment. *Journal of Pediatric Psychology, 16,* 643–663.

Gottlieb, B. H. (1983). Social support strategies: Guidelines for mental health practice. Beverly Hills: Sage.

Grand, S. D., & Strohmer, D. C. (1983). Minority perception of the disabled. *Rehabilitation Counseling Bulletin, 27,* 117–119.

Griffith, J. (1985). Social support providers: Who are they? Where are they met? and the Relationship of network characteristics to psychological distress. *Basic and Applied Social Psychology, 6,* 41–60.

Hackett, G., & Betz, N. (1996). Self-efficacy and career choice and development. In J. E. Maddux (Ed.), *Self-efficacy, adaption and adjustment.* New York: Plenum.

Hale-Benson, J. (1986). Black children: Their roots, culture, and learning styles. Baltimore, MD: Johns Hopkins University Press.

Hanson, S., Buckelew, S. P., Hewett, J., & O'Neal, G. (1993). The relationship between coping and adjustment after spinal cord injury: A 5-year follow-up study. *Rehabilitation Psychology, 38,* 41–52.

Hayden, G. T., & Gehlback, S. N. (1983). The epidemiologic evidence for a relationship between social support and health. *Journal of Epidemiology, 117,* 521–537.

Herbert, J. T., & Cheatham, H. E. (1988). Africentricity and the Black disability experience: A theoretical orientation for rehabilitation counselors. *Journal of Applied Rehabilitation Counseling, 19,* 50–54.

Hoffman, H. R., & Loring, K. (1992). Self-efficacy expectancies in chronic obstructive pulmonary disease rehabilitation. In R. Schwarzer (Ed.), *Self-efficacy: Thought control of action.* Washington, DC: Hemisphere Publishing Corporation.

Hornor, L. L. (1995). *Black Americans: A Statistical Sourcebook.* Palo Alto, CA: Information Publications.

Hughes, M., & Demo, D. V. (1989). Self-perceptions of Black Americans: Self-esteem and personal efficacy. *American Journal of Sociology, 95,* 132–159.

Hunt, J. G., & Hunt, L. L. (1977). Racial inequality and self-image: Identity maintenance and identity diffusion. *Sociology and Social Research, 61,* 539–559.

Institute of Medicine. (1991). *Disability in America.* Washington, DC: National Academy Press.

Jensen, M. P., Turner, J. A., & Romano, J. M. (1991). Self-efficacy and outcome expectancies: Relationship to chronic pain coping strategies and adjustment. *Rehabilitation Medicine, 44,* 263–269.

Jones, J. M. (1997). *Prejudice and Racism.* New York: McGraw-Hill.

Kalinsky, E. M., Rubison, L., Lawrence, L., & Levy, S. R. (1990). AIDS, runaways, and self-efficacy. *Family and Community Health, 13,* 65–72.

Karenga, M. (1977). *Kwanzaa: Origin, concepts, practice.* Los Angeles: Kawaida Publishers.

Kessler, R. C., & McLeod, J. P. (1985). Social support and mental health in community samples. In S. Cohen & S. L. Syme (Eds), *Social Support and Health* (pp. 219–240). Orlando, FL: Academic Press.

Kroeber, A. L., & Cluckholm, C. (1963). *Culture: A critical review of concepts and definitions.* New York: Vintage.

Landrine, H., & Klonoff, E. A. (1995). *African American Acculturation.* Thousand Oaks, CA: Sage.

Landrine, H., & Klonoff, E. A. (1992). Culture and health-related schemas: A review and proposal for interdisciplinary integration. *Health Psychology, 11,* 267–276.

Lazarus, R. S., & Folkman, S. (1984). Stress, appraisal and coping. New York: Springer.

Leininger, M. (1978). *Transcultural nursing: Concepts, theories, and practices.* New York: Wiley.

Lewis, D., Belgrave, F. Z., & Scott, R. B. (1990). Patient adherence in minority populations. In S. Shumaker, E. Schron, and J. K. Ockene (Eds.), *The adoption and maintenance of behaviors for optimal health.* New York: Springer.

Maddux, J. E. (1996). *Self-efficacy, adaptation, and adjustment.* New York: Plenum.

Maddux, J. E., & Lewis, J. (1995). Self-efficacy and adjustment: Basic principles and issues. In J. E. Maddux (ed.), *Self-efficacy, adaptation, and adjustment.* New York: Plenum.

Maier, S. F., Watkins, L. R., & Flesher, M. (1994). Psychoimmuneurology. *American Psychologist, 49,* 1004–1017.

Manton, K. B., Patrick, C. H. & Johnson, K. W. (1987). Health differentials between Blacks and Whites: Recent trends in mortality and morbidity. *Milbank Quarterly, 65,* 129–199.

Martin, E., & Martin, J. M. (1978). *The Black extended family.* Chicago: University of Chicago Press.

McAdoo, H. P. (1981). *Black families.* Beverly Hills, CA: Sage.

McAdoo, H. P. (1993). *Family ethnicity: Strength in diversity.* Newbury Park, CA: Sage.

McAdoo, H. P. (1982). Stress-absorbing systems in Black families. *Family Relations, 31,* 479–488.

McNeil, J. M. (1993). Americans with disabilities: 1991–1992. U.S. Bureau of the Census. Current Population Reports. Washington, DC: Government Printing Office.

Mindel, C. H. (1980). Extended familism among urban Mexican Americans, Anglos, and Blacks. *Hispanic Journal of Behavioral Sciences,* 1980, *2,* 21–34.

Mindel, C. H., & Wright, R. (1982). The use of social services by Black and White elderly: The role of social support systems. *Journal of Gerontological Social Work, 4,* 107–125.

Mitchell, J. K., Brodwin, M. G., & Benoit, R. B. (1990). Strengthening the workers' compensation system by increasing client efficacy. *Journal of Applied Rehabilitation Counseling, 21,* 22–26.

Murdock, G. P. (1989). *Theories of illness: A world survey.* Pittsburgh, PA: University of Pittsburgh Press.

Myers, H. F. (1982). Stress, ethnicity, and social class: A model for research with Black populations. In E. Jones & S. Korchin (Eds.), *Minority Mental Health.* New York: Praeger.

Myers, L. J. (1988). *An Afrocentric world-view: Introduction to an optimal psychology.* Dubuque, IA: Quintal-Hunt.

Neighbors, H. W., & Jackson, J. S. (1984). The use of informal and formal help: Four patterns of illness behavior in the Black community. *American Journal of Community Psychology, 12,* 629–644.

Neighbors, H. W., Jackson, J. S., Bowman, P., & Gurin, G. (1983). Stress, coping and black mental health: Preliminary findings from a national study. *Prevention in Human Services, 2*, 979–983.

Nobles, W. W. (1986). *African psychology: Towards its reclamation, reascension, and revitalization*. Oakland, CA: Black Family Institute.

Nobles, W. W. (1990). African philosophy: Foundations of Black psychology. In R. L. Jones (Ed.), *Black Psychology*. Berkeley, CA: Cobb & Henry.

Nwanze, H., & Sowemino, G. (1987). Maternal stress, superstition and communicative behavior with Nigerian cleft lip and palate children. *Scandinavian Journal of Plastic Reconstructive Surgery, 21*, 15–18.

O'Leary, A., Shoor, S., Lorig, K., & Holman, H. R. (1988). A cognitive-behavioral treatment for rheumatoid arthritis. *Health Psychology, 7*, 527–544.

Partridge, C., & Johnson, M. (1989). Perceived control of recovery from physical disability: Measurement and prediction. *British Journal Clinical Psychology, 28*, 53–59.

Phillips, F. B. (1990). NTU psychotherapy: An Afrocentric approach. *Journal of Black Psychology, 17*, 55–74.

Phillips, G. Y. (1996). Stress and residential well-being. In H. W. & J. S. Jackson (Eds.), *Mental Health in Black America*. Thousand Oaks, CA: Sage.

Rackley, R. (1994). Selected parental and child characteristics as predictors of coping strategies and social support among African-American families with disabilities. Unpublished doctoral dissertation, Howard University, Washington, DC, 1994.

Randolph, S. M., & Banks, H. D. (1993). Making a way out of no way: The promise of Africentric approaches to HIV prevention. *Journal of Black Psychology, 19*, 204–214.

Raymond, J. S., Rhoads, D. L., & Raymond, R. I. (1980). The relative impact of family and social involvement on Chicano mental health. *American Journal of Community Psychology, 8*, 557–569.

Rosenberg, M. J. (1965). *Society and the adolescent self-image*. Princeton, NJ: Princeton University Press.

Rotter, J. B. (1966). Generalized expectancies for internal versus external control of reinforcement. *Psychological Monographs, 80*, 1–28.

Sackett, D. L., & Snow, J. C. (1979). The magnitude of compliance and noncompliance. In R. B. Haynes, D. W. Taylor, & D. L. Sackett (Eds.), *Compliance in health care* (pp. 11–22). Baltimore, MD: Johns Hopkins University Press.

Schiaffino, K. M., & Revenson, T. A. (1992). The role of perceived self-efficacy, perceived control, and causal attributions in adaptation to rheumatoid arthritis: Distinguishing mediator from moderator effects. *Personality and Social Psychology Bulletin, 18*, 709–718.

Schiaffino, K. M., Revenson, T. A., & Gibofsky, A. (1991). Assessing the impact of self-efficacy beliefs on adaptation to rheumatoid arthritics. *Arthritis Care and Research, 4*, 150–157.

Schumaker, S. A., & Brownell, A. (1984). Toward a theory of social support: Closing conceptual gaps. *Journal of Social Issues, 40*, 11–36.

Smith-Ruiz, D. (1985). Relationship between depression, social support, and physical illness among elderly Blacks: Research notes. *Journal of the National Medical Association, 77*, 1017–1019.

Stephens, D. (1985). Perception of pregnancy and social support as predictors of alcohol consumption during pregnancy. *Alcoholism-Clinical/Experimental Research, 9*, 344–348.

Stroebe, W., & Stroebo, M. (1997). The social psychology of social support. In E. T. Higgins & A. W. Kruglanski (Eds.), *Social psychology: Handbook of basic principles*. New York: Gilford.

Stretcher, V. J., DeVellis, B. M., Becker, M. H., & Rosenstock, I. M. (1986). The role of self-efficacy in achieving health behavior change. *Health Education Quarterly, 13*, 79–93.

Strogatz, D. S., and James, S. A. (1986). Social support and hypertension among Blacks and Whites in a rural, southern community. *American Journal of Epidemiology*, 1986, *124*, 949–956.

Taal, E., Rasker, J., Seydel, E., & Weigman, O. (1993). Health status, adherence with health recommendations, self-efficacy and social support in patients with rheumatoid arthritis. *Patient Education and Counseling, 20*, 63–76.

Taylor, R. J., & Chatters, L. M. (1986). Patterns of informal support to elderly Black adults: Family, friends, and church members. *Social Work, 31*, 432–436.

Taylor, S. E. (1991). *Health psychology*. New York: McGraw-Hill.

Taylor, S. E., Locke, E. A., Lee, C., & Gist, M. E. (1984). Behavior and faculty research productivity: What are the mechanisms? *Organizational Behavior and Human Performance, 34*, 402–418.

Terry, D. J. (1992). Stress, coping, and coping resources as correlates of adaptation in myocardial infarction patients. *British Journal of Clinical Psychology, 31*, 215–225.

Thomas, V. G., Milburn, N. G., Brown, D. R., & Gary, L. E. (1988). Social support and depressive symptoms among blacks. *Journal of Black Psychology, 14*, 35–45.

Thompson, R. J., Gil, K. M., Abrams, M. R., & Phillips, G. (1992). Stress, coping, and psychological adjustment of adults with sickle cell disease. *Journal of Consulting and Clinical Psychology, 60*, 433–440.

Thompson, S., & Spacapan, S. (1991). Perceived control in vulnerable populations. *Journal of Social Issues, 47*, 1–20.

Toliver-Weddington, G. (1990). Cultural considerations in the treatment of craniofacial malformations in African Americans. *Cleft Palate Journal, 27*, 289–293.

Tyler, F. (1978). Individual psychosocial competence: A personality configuration. *Education and Psychological Measurements, 38*, 309–323.

U.S. Department of Health and Human Services (1990). Health Status of the Disadvantaged: Chart Book. Washington, DC: U.S. Government Printing Office.

U.S. Department of Health and Human Services (1986). Report of the Secretary's Task Force on Black and Minority Health. Washington DC: US. Government Printing Office.

Varni, J. W., Setoguchi, Y., Rappaport, L. R., & Talbot, D. (1992). Psychological adjustment and perceived social support in children with congenital/acquired limb deficiencies. *Journal of Behavioral Medicine, 15*, 31–44.

Varni, J. W., Wilcox, K. T., & Hanson, V. (1988). Mediating effects of family social support on child psychological adjustment in juvenile rheumatoid arthritis. *Health Psychology, 7*, 421–431.

Walker, S., & Asbury, C. (1993). *The Walker/Asbury structured interview system.* Questionnaire available from the Howard University Research Training Center for Access to Rehabilitation and Economic Opportunity, 2900 Van Ness Street, N.W., Washington, DC.

Walker, S., & Belgrave, F. Z. (1995). Coping patterns among families with children with disabilities (Technical report). Washington, DC: Howard University, Research and Training Center for Access to Rehabilitation and Economic Opportunity, 2900 Van Ness Street, N.W.

Walker, S., Belgrave, F. Z., Jarama, S. L., Ukawuilulu, J., & Rackley, R. (1995). The effectiveness of a support group intervention for increasing employment efficacy for ethnic minorities with disabilities. Unpublished manuscript.

Walker, S., Belgrave, F. Z., Roberts, V., & Palmer, R. (1986). *Status of the Black disabled in the rehabilitation system.* Research report of the National Survey of the Howard University Rehabilitation Project. Washington, DC: Howard University Center for the Study of Handicapped Children and Adults.

Walker, S., Saravanabhavan, R. C., Williams P., Brown, O., & West, T. (1996). An examination of the impact of federally supported community services and educational systems on underserved people with disabilities from diverse cultural populations. Washington, DC: Howard University Research and Training Center for Access to Rehabilitation and Economic Opportunity.

Wallander, J. L., Feldman, W. S., & Varni, J. W. (1989). Physical status and psychosocial adjustment in children with spina bifida. *Journal of Pediatric Psychology, 14*, 89–102.

Wallander, J. L., & Varni, J. W. (1989). Social support and adjustment in chronically ill and handicapped children. *American Journal of Community Psychology, 17*, 185–201.

Wallander, J. L., Varni, J. W., Babani, L., Banis, H. T., & Wilcox, K. T. (1989). Family resources as resistance factors for psychological maladjustment in chronically ill and handicapped children. *Journal of Pediatric Psychology, 14*, 157–173.

Wassen, R. (1992). Self-efficacy as a predictor of adjustment to multiple sclerosis. *Journal of Neuroscience Nursing, 24*, 224–229.

Weitzel, H. H., & Waller, P. R. (1990). Predictive factors for health promotive behaviors in White, Hispanic, and Black blue-collar workers. *Family and Community Health, 13*, 23–24.

Wilson, M. E. (1988). Critical factors in the employment success of Black Americans with disabilities. In S. Walker et al. (Eds.), *Building Bridges to Independence.* Proceedings of a national conference sponsored by the Center for the Study of Handicapped Children and Youth and the President's Committee on Employment of People with Disabilities.

Wilson, M. N. (1989). Child development in the context of the Black extended family. *American Psychologist, 44*, 380–385.

Wright, B. A. (1960). *Physical disability: A psychological approach.* (2nd ed.). New York: Harper and Row.

Yuker, H. E. (1994). Variables that influence attitudes toward people with disabilities: Conclusions from the data. *Journal of Social Behavior and Personality, 9*, 3–22.

Zea, M. C., Belgrave, F. Z., Townsend, T., Jarama, S. L., & Banks, S. (1996). The influence of social support and active coping on depression among African Americans and Latinos with disabilities. *Journal of Rehabilitation Psychology, 41*, 225–241

Index

About the Author

FAYE Z. BELGRAVE is a professor in the Department of Psychology at Virginia Commonwealth University in Richmond, Virginia.

ISBN 0-86569-242-4
90000>
EAN
9 780865 692428
HARDCOVER BAR CODE